03/22

DIABETES

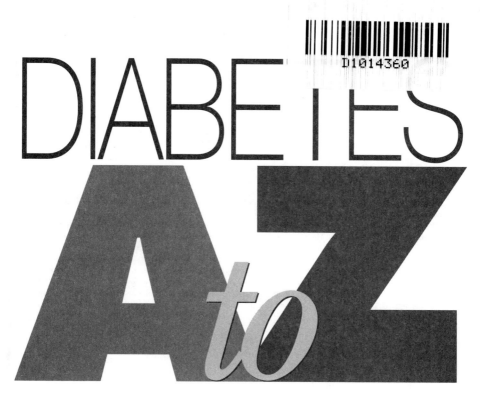

A to Z

What You Need to Know
About Diabetes – Simply Put

Fifth Edition

▲. American Diabetes Association.

Cure • Care • Commitment℠

Director, Book Publishing, John Fedor; *Associate Director, Consumer Books,* Sherrye Landrum; *Editor,* Abe Ogden; *Associate Director, Book Production,* Peggy M. Rote; *Composition,* Circle Graphics; *Cover Design,* Koncept Inc.; *Printer,* Port City Press.

Printed in the United States of America
7 9 10 8 6

The suggestions and information contained in this publication are generally consistent with the *Clinical Practice Recommendations* and other policies of the American Diabetes Association, but they do not represent the policy or position of the Association or any of its boards or committees. Reasonable steps have been taken to ensure the accuracy of the information presented. However, the American Diabetes Association cannot ensure the safety or efficacy of any product or service described in this publication. Individuals are advised to consult a physician or other appropriate health care professional before undertaking any diet or exercise program or taking any medication referred to in this publication. Professionals must use and apply their own professional judgment, experience, and training and should not rely solely on the information contained in this publication before prescribing any diet, exercise, or medication. The American Diabetes Association—its officers, directors, employees, volunteers, and members—assumes no responsibility or liability for personal or other injury, loss, or damage that may result from the suggestions or information in this publication.

∞ The paper in this publication meets the requirements of the ANSI Standard Z39.48-1992 (permanence of paper).

ADA titles may be purchased for business or promotional use or for special sales. To purchase this book in large quantities, or for custom editions of this book with your logo, contact Lee Romano Sequeira, Special Sales & Promotions, at the address below, or at LRomano@diabetes.org or 703-299-2046.

American Diabetes Association
1701 North Beauregard Street
Alexandria, Virginia 22311

Library of Congress Cataloging-in-Publication Data

Diabetes A to Z : what you need to know about diabetes, simply put.—5th ed.
   p. cm.
  Includes index.
  ISBN 1-58040-183-X (alk. paper)
  1. Diabetes—Popular works. I. American Diabetes Association

RC660.4.D526 2003
616.4'62—dc21

                2003056267

Table of Contents

Foreword

Maybe you've just been diagnosed with diabetes or maybe you've had diabetes for years. Perhaps a member of your family or a friend has diabetes. Whatever your situation, you want to find out all you can about the disease. That's where *Diabetes A to Z* can help. It explains everything you need to know about diabetes in clear, simple terms.

Diabetes A to Z is an encyclopedia of diabetes. It is arranged alphabetically, so you can more easily find the information you need. You may also enjoy just browsing from entry to entry.

The information in each entry will help you understand how to balance your diabetes care with a full and active lifestyle. You will even find helpful tips on coping with the social and emotional challenges of day-to-day life with diabetes.

We hope *Diabetes A to Z* helps you understand your diabetes better, so that you can live a longer, happier, and healthier life.

Frank Vinicor, MD, MPH
Past President, American Diabetes Association

Acknowledgments

Many thanks to the reviewers of this edition:

Robert M. Anderson, EdD

Charlotte A. Hayes, CDE, MS, MSc, RD

Morey W. Haymond, MD

Crystal Jackson, Shereen Arent, Michael Mawby, Holly Whelan, and Tom Boyer

David S. Schade, MD

Clara Schneider, MS, RD, RN, LD, CDE

Virginia Valentine, CNS, BC-ADM, CDE

Donald K. Zettervall, RPh, CDE

A1C Test

Hemoglobin is a protein inside red blood cells. Hemoglobin carries oxygen from the lungs to all the cells of the body.

Like other proteins, hemoglobin can join with sugars, such as glucose. When this happens, it becomes glycated hemoglobin, referred to as A1C (or sometimes as HbA1c).

The more glucose there is in the blood, the more hemoglobin will join with it. Once joined, hemoglobin and glucose stay that way for the life of the red blood cell—about 4 months.

The A1C test measures the amount of glycohemoglobin in your red blood cells. The A1C test is usually done by a lab.

A sample of your blood is taken. The blood can be taken at any time of the day. It does not matter what food you last ate. It does not matter what your blood glucose level is at the time of the test.

WHAT THE A1C TEST CAN DO

- Tell you about your blood glucose level for the past 2 to 3 months. You can then see how your blood glucose control has been.

- Allow you to compare the A1C test results with blood glucose checks you have done yourself or tests your doctor has done. If the tests do not agree, you may need to change the way you check or when you check.

- Help you judge whether your diabetes care plan is working. If your long-term blood glucose level is high, something in your plan may need to be changed.
- Show you how a change in your plan has affected your diabetes. Perhaps you started to exercise more. An A1C test can confirm the good effects exercise has had on your blood glucose control.

WHAT THE NUMBERS MEAN

There is more than one way to measure A1C. And there is more than one kind of A1C. One kind of A1C may be measured by several different tests. Because of this, A1C tests done at different labs may give different numbers.

If you change doctors or your doctor changes labs, be sure to find out what the numbers from the new lab mean. Usually, the higher the A1C test number, the higher the blood glucose levels. Work with your health care team to set A1C goals.

WHEN TO GET AN A1C TEST

Have an A1C test done when you find out you have diabetes. After that, have the test done at least 2–4 times a year.

WHY KEEP DOING SELF-CHECKS OF BLOOD GLUCOSE?

The A1C test can't replace the checks you do each day to measure the level of glucose in your blood (see Blood Glucose, Self-Checks). Self-checks help you decide how to treat diabetes at that moment. What you do to keep daily blood glucose levels in range will show up in your A1C test results.

Activity

ctivity is good for everyone, especially people with diabetes. Activity makes your insulin work harder and faster, which means you may need less insulin or diabetes pills to control your diabetes. Moderate activity lowers your risk of heart disease, high blood pressure, and may reduce your risk for colon cancer. It can improve your blood fat levels, reduce your body fat, and help you lose weight.

Activity keeps your joints, muscles, and bones healthy and can make them stronger. And activity can increase your energy; relieve symptoms of depression, anxiety, and stress; and improve your mood. In short, activity could help you have a longer, happier, healthier life.

So go ahead. Get up on your feet and move around. When you are on your feet and moving around, you use two to three times more energy than when you sit.

WAYS TO GET MOVING

- Get up to change TV channels instead of using the remote.
- Do the ironing while watching TV.
- Walk around your house during TV commercials.
- Wash dishes, load the dishwasher, or load the clothes washer or dryer during commercials.
- Mop the kitchen floor.
- Vacuum the living room.

- Sweep your sidewalk.
- Wash and wax your car.
- Use a rake instead of a leaf blower.
- Use a push lawn mower instead of an electric one.
- Plant and maintain an herb or vegetable garden.
- Take your pet for a walk.
- Push your baby in a stroller.
- Play actively with children.
- Volunteer to work for a school or hospital.
- Walk to the subway or bus stop.
- Take the stairs instead of the elevator or escalator.
- Stand or walk around while you're on the phone.
- Walk during lunch, during your break, while the oven is preheating, or while waiting for your prescription.
- Run errands that require walking, such as grocery shopping.
- Park your car farther away from your destination.
- Take a walk with someone you want to talk with.

Be sure to check with your doctor before increasing your level of physical activity. If you have not been active lately, start with just 5 to 10 minutes of an activity and work up to longer or harder activity sessions.

Alcohol

One or two drinks a day will have little effect on your blood glucose level if you have good control of your diabetes, are free of complications, and drink the alcohol close to or with a meal. But drinking two drinks on an empty stomach can cause low blood glucose if you are taking certain diabetes pills or insulin or if you were just exercising or about to exercise.

ALCOHOL AND LOW BLOOD GLUCOSE

Insulin lowers your blood glucose. Certain diabetes pills (sulfonylureas, meglitinides, and D-phenylalanines) make your body release more insulin to lower blood glucose. Exercise makes your insulin work better at lowering blood glucose.

Usually, if your blood glucose drops too low, the liver puts more glucose into the blood. (The liver has its own supply of glucose, called glycogen.) But when alcohol, a toxin, is in the body, the liver wants to get rid of it first. While the liver is taking care of the alcohol, it may let blood glucose drop to dangerous levels.

How to avoid low blood glucose

- Always eat something with carbohydrate when you drink alcohol.
- Check your blood glucose before, during, and after drinking. Alcohol can lower blood glucose as long as 8 to 12 hours after your last drink.

- Follow the *Dietary Guidelines for Americans* recommendation of no more than two drinks per day for men and no more than one drink per day for women. A drink equals a 12 oz beer, 5 oz wine, or 1.5 oz liquor.

If you have low blood glucose after you drink, people might smell the alcohol and think you are drunk. The signs are the same. Tell them you have low blood glucose. Tell them what they need to do to help you take care of it. Wear a medical I.D. bracelet stating that you have diabetes. This will help in case you can't talk.

If you drink and then drive when you have low blood glucose, you may be pulled over for drunk driving. You may even have an accident. When you drink—even a small amount—let someone else drive. Pick a responsible person ahead of time.

ALCOHOL AND COMPLICATIONS

Alcohol can worsen nerve damage, eye diseases, high blood pressure, and high blood fats. If you have any of these problems, ask your health care provider how much alcohol, if any, is safe for you to drink.

ALCOHOL AND YOUR MEAL PLAN

Work with a dietitian to include your favorite drink in your meal plan. Be aware that regular beer, sweet wines, and wine coolers will raise your blood glucose more than light beer, dry wines, and liquors (such as vodka, scotch, and whiskey) because they contain more carbohydrate. Carbohydrate is the main nutrient that raises blood glucose.

If you are watching your weight, be aware that alcoholic drinks can have anywhere from 60 to 300 calories each. Just cutting down on the number of drinks or changing the type of drink can help with weight loss.

How to cut calories

- Use 80 proof in place of 100 proof alcohol. The lower the proof number, the less alcohol in the liquor. Each gram of alcohol has 7 calories.

- Put less liquor in your drink.
- Use no-calorie mixers, such as diet soda, club soda, or water.
- Choose light beer over regular beer.
- Choose dry wine over sweet or fruity wines and wine coolers.
- Try a wine spritzer made with a small amount of wine and a lot of club soda.

Drink	Serving	Calories	Exchanges
Liquor	1.5 oz	107	2 Fats
Table wine	5.0 oz	100	2 Fats
Wine cooler	12 oz	196	3 Fats, 1 Starch
Regular beer	12 oz	151	2 Fats, 1 Starch
Light beer	12 oz	97	2 Fats

COOKING WITH ALCOHOL

When alcohol is heated in cooking, either on top of the stove or in the oven, some of it evaporates. How much of it evaporates depends on how long you cook it. If you cook it for 30 minutes or less, about one-third of the alcohol calories will remain. You'll need to count them in your meal plan. If you use alcohol regularly (3 times a week) in your cooking, the calories can add up.

Blood Glucose

The foods you eat are broken down into glucose by your body. Glucose is a sugar. Glucose travels through your blood to your cells. Cells use glucose for energy. To get inside your cells, glucose needs the help of insulin.

In people with diabetes, there is a problem with the insulin. Sometimes there is no insulin (see Type 1 Diabetes). Other times there is insulin, but the body has trouble using it or there isn't enough of it (see Type 2 Diabetes).

When insulin is not able to do its job, glucose cannot get into the cells. Instead, glucose collects in the blood. The amount of glucose in your blood is called your blood glucose level.

Too much glucose in the blood is called hyperglycemia or high blood glucose. Too little glucose in the blood is called hypoglycemia or low blood glucose. Blood glucose that has gone up too far or down too low can make you feel ill and harm your body (see Blood Glucose, High; Blood Glucose, Low).

To feel good and stay healthy, keep your blood glucose between the highs and lows—in a range your doctor advises. See the table on the next page.

Keeping your blood glucose in range and avoiding the highs and lows takes some effort. You can do it by balancing food, activity, and diabetes pills or insulin. One of your best tools is a blood glucose meter. Here are some tips for success.

PLASMA BLOOD GLUCOSE RANGES FOR PEOPLE WITH DIABETES

Time	Glucose (mg/dl)
In the morning, before breakfast	90 to 130
Before meals	90 to 130
2 hours after a meal	Under 180

These ranges are based on blood glucose checks you do at home (see Blood Glucose, Self-Checks) rather than lab tests. These may not be the best ranges for you. Talk to your health care team about what your ranges should be.

FOOD

- Follow your meal plan (see Meal Planning).
- Include snacks in your meal plan only if your diabetes care provider or dietitian recommends it.
- Eat meals and snacks around the same times each day.
- Don't skip or delay meals or snacks.
- Eat the same amounts of foods from day to day.
- If you take insulin, ask your diabetes care provider how to adjust your dose when you want to eat more or less than usual.

ACTIVITY

- Follow your exercise program.
- If you take insulin or certain diabetes pills (the sulfonylureas, the meglitinides) and if you are going to exercise for more than 1 hour, you may need to eat snacks. Examples of snacks are a piece of fruit, 1/2 cup of juice, 1/2 bagel, or a small roll. Talk with a dietitian or diabetes educator about how much and when to eat.
- Be sure to check your blood glucose levels after exercise. Exercise lowers blood glucose for as long as 10 to 24 hours afterward.

- If you take insulin, ask your diabetes care provider if you need to adjust your dose for exercise.

DIABETES PILLS OR INSULIN

- Take insulin or diabetes pills as your doctor has directed.
- Talk with your doctor about changing your insulin or diabetes pills if your blood glucose levels are not in your range. Perhaps a different dose or type of insulin or pills would work better for you.
- If you take insulin, ask your diabetes care provider about the best places to inject it. Some people find that taking their insulin in the same place keeps blood glucose steadier.
- Consider an insulin pump. Pumps imitate the natural release of insulin better than injections do (see Insulin Pumps).

CHECKING BLOOD GLUCOSE

- Check your blood glucose often. If you check once a day, consider two or three times a day.
- Check your blood glucose more often if:
  - You ate too much or too little food or tried a new food
  - You delayed or skipped a meal or snack
  - You are sick
  - You are under stress
  - You did not take your insulin or diabetes pills
  - You took too much insulin
  - You took too many diabetes pills
  - You did not do your usual exercise
  - You exercised harder or longer than usual

Blood Glucose, High

Too much glucose in the blood is called hyperglycemia or high blood glucose. High blood glucose is one of the signs of diabetes. Over time, high blood glucose can damage your eyes, kidneys, heart, nerves, and blood vessels.

CAUSES OF HIGH BLOOD GLUCOSE

- You ate too much food.
- You ate too much carbohydrate.
- You took too little insulin.
- You did not take your insulin.
- You took too few diabetes pills.
- You did not take your diabetes pills.
- You are sick.
- You feel stressed.
- You skipped your usual exercise or activity.

High blood glucose is harder to sense than low blood glucose. If your glucose is very high, you may feel some of the following signs.

SIGNS OF HIGH BLOOD GLUCOSE

- Headache
- Blurry vision

- Thirst
- Hunger
- Upset stomach
- Frequent urination
- Dry, itchy skin

You may not be able to tell that your glucose is too high by these signs alone. The only sure way to know is to check your blood glucose (see Blood Glucose, Self-Checks). Your glucose reading will help you decide what to do.

HOW TO TREAT HIGH BLOOD GLUCOSE

If your blood glucose is between 180 and 250 mg/dl

1. Do as your doctor has advised you. You may have been told to try one of the following:
   - A small extra dose of regular (short-acting) insulin
   - A smaller upcoming snack
2. Check your blood glucose again after 1–2 hours.

If your blood glucose stays above 250 mg/dl

Check for signs of diabetic ketoacidosis (see Urine Ketone Test) or hyperglycemic hyperosmolar nonketotic state (see HHS). If you have any of the signs, call your doctor right away.

If your blood glucose stays above 350 mg/dl

Call your doctor.

If your blood glucose stays above 500 mg/dl

Call your doctor and have someone take you to a hospital emergency room right away.

Blood Glucose, Low

Too little glucose in the blood is called hypoglycemia or low blood glucose. Low blood glucose may occur if you use insulin or take certain diabetes pills (the sulfonylureas, the meglitinides). If not treated, low blood glucose can make you pass out. At worst, low blood glucose may cause seizures, coma, and even death.

CAUSES OF LOW BLOOD GLUCOSE

- You ate too little food.
- You ate too few carbohydrates.
- You delayed a meal or snack.
- You skipped a meal or snack.
- You exercised harder or longer than usual.
- You were more active than usual.
- You took too much insulin or too many diabetes pills.
- You drank alcohol on an empty stomach.

WARNING SIGNS OF LOW BLOOD GLUCOSE

There are many warning signs of low blood glucose. Your own signs may be different from what someone else feels.

Learn your early warning signs of low blood glucose. Share your signs with someone who can help you notice them.

WARNING SIGNS

Your signs may not be on this list.

Angry	Irritable	Sick to stomach
Anxious	Light-headed	Sleepy
Clammy	Nervous	Stubborn
Clumsy	Numb	Sweaty
Confused	Pale	Tense
Hungry	Sad	Tired
Impatient	Shaky	Weak

You may also have blurry vision, a dry mouth, a headache, or a pounding heart. When any of your warning signs occur, you need to treat low blood glucose right away.

HOW TO TREAT YOURSELF FOR LOW BLOOD GLUCOSE

1. Check your blood glucose with a meter if you can (see Blood Glucose, Self-Checks).

   If your blood glucose is under 70 mg/dl

   Go to steps 2 and 3. If you can't check, go to steps 2 and 4.

2. Eat or drink something with about 15 grams (1/2 oz) of carbohydrate. Foods with 15 grams of carbohydrate are listed in the table on the next page.

3. Wait 15 to 20 minutes, then check again.

   If your blood glucose is still below 70 mg/dl

   Repeat steps 2 and 3. If you have repeated steps 2 and 3 and your blood glucose is still below 70 mg/dl, call your doctor or have someone take you to a hospital emergency room. You may need help to treat your low blood glucose. Or something else may be causing the signs.

If your blood glucose is over 70 mg/dl

Stop drinking and/or eating foods listed in the table. You may still feel the signs of low blood glucose even after your blood glucose is back up. Go to step 4.

4. If your next meal is more than an hour away, eat a small snack of carbohydrate and protein. Try a slice of bread with reduced-fat peanut butter or six crackers with low-fat cheese.

TREAT LOW BLOOD GLUCOSE WITH ONE OF THESE FOODS

Glucose tablets or gel (dose is printed on the package)

1/3 cup (4 oz) of fruit juice

1/3 can (4 oz) of a regular (not sugar-free) soft drink

1 cup (8 oz) of fat-free milk

2 tablespoons of raisins (40 to 50)

3 graham crackers

1 tablespoon of granulated sugar

6 saltine crackers

1 tablespoon of honey or syrup

HOW TO HAVE SOMEONE ELSE TREAT YOUR LOW BLOOD GLUCOSE

Sometimes you will not be able to treat low blood glucose yourself. Maybe you do not notice your signs. Or maybe low blood glucose has made you too confused to treat yourself. Whatever the reason, teach someone else ahead of time to do it.

Keep foods to treat low blood glucose near you at all times. Place a small box of juice in your desk drawer at work or at school. Put glucose tablets or gel in your purse or coat pocket and in the glove compartment of your car. Tell others where you keep them.

If you take insulin, get a glucagon emergency kit. Your doctor can prescribe one. Glucagon is a hormone that is made in the pancreas. Glucagon makes the liver release glucose into the blood and shuts down insulin release.

A glucagon kit comes with a syringe of glucagon and instructions on how to use it. Keep the kit with you. Tell family, friends, and coworkers where you keep it. You or a member of your health care team can teach them how to use it.

If you can swallow

1. Have someone get you to eat or drink something with carbohydrate in it.

If you cannot swallow or if you pass out

1. Have someone inject you with glucagon in the front of the thigh or the shoulder muscle.

2. Have someone turn you on your side. This will keep you from choking if you throw up from the glucagon. (Some people feel sick to their stomach after glucagon.)

3. Once you are alert, eat a snack of carbohydrate that's easy on your stomach. Try six saltine crackers. Follow it up with a snack of protein, such as a slice of turkey breast or low-fat cheese.

4. Check your blood glucose every 30 to 60 minutes to make sure low blood glucose is not coming back.

If you cannot swallow and glucagon is not available OR
If you cannot swallow and nobody knows how to use glucagon

1. Have someone call 911 for an ambulance.

2. Have someone moisten his or her fingertip, dip the fingertip in table sugar, and rub the sugar-coated fingertip against the inside of your cheek until the sugar dissolves, being careful to keep the finger away from your teeth. (If you go into a seizure, you may bite the finger.)

OR

Have someone open a tube of glucose gel or cake frosting and insert the open end inside your cheek. Have the person squeeze a small amount of the gel or frosting into your mouth and massage the outside of your cheek.

Keep doing step 2 until the ambulance arrives.

Blood Glucose, Self-Checks

Self-checks are those you do yourself. A blood glucose self-check tells you how much glucose is in your blood at any one time. Anyone with diabetes can benefit from self-checks.

WHY CHECK BLOOD GLUCOSE?

When you found out you had diabetes, you and your health care team worked out a diabetes care plan. The plan was set up to help you keep your blood glucose levels in your range (see Blood Glucose). Your plan may include healthy eating, regular exercise or activity, insulin, or diabetes pills.

One of the best ways to keep track of how well your diabetes care plan is working is to check your blood glucose. Checking helps you find out what happens to your blood glucose level when you eat certain foods, do certain exercises or activities, or lose weight. Checking helps you find out what happens to your blood glucose level when you take insulin or diabetes pills, are sick, or are under stress.

A blood glucose check can help you decide how to take care of your diabetes. It may prompt you to eat a snack, take more insulin, or exercise more. It may alert you to treat high or low blood glucose.

HOW TO CHECK BLOOD GLUCOSE

You can check your blood glucose with either a glucose meter or a test strip that you read by eye. It's important to follow the instructions that come with the product you buy. Most glu-cose self-checks go as follows:

1. Wash your hands with soap and water. Dry them.
2. Prick the side of your finger with a lancet.
3. Squeeze out a drop of blood.
4. Let the drop of blood fall on a test strip pad, if possible.
5. Insert the test strip into your glucose meter.
6. Read your blood glucose number in the window on the meter.
7. Dispose of the lancet the same way as your syringe needles.
8. Record your finding.

WHEN TO CHECK BLOOD GLUCOSE

Your diabetes care provider can help you figure out when to check your blood glucose. Checking at specific times can be useful. For instance, a check done 1 or 2 hours after a meal lets you see how high your blood glucose rises after you eat certain kinds and amounts of foods. A check at 2 or 3 A.M. tells you whether you have low blood glucose at night. There are eight possible check times:

1. Before breakfast
2. 1 to 2 hours after breakfast
3. Before lunch
4. 1 to 2 hours after lunch
5. Before supper
6. 1 to 2 hours after supper
7. Before bedtime
8. At 2 or 3 A.M.

The more you check, the more you will know about your blood glu-cose levels. And the more you know about your blood glucose levels, the better able you will be to get those levels in your range. Here are some check times to talk about with your health care team.

If you have type 1 diabetes

Check before each meal and at bedtime every day.

If you have type 2 diabetes and are on insulin

Check two to four times a day. Vary the times you check.

If you have type 2 diabetes and are taking diabetes pills

Check one or two times a day. If you check once a day, do it before you eat breakfast. If you check twice a day, check first when you get up in the morning. Vary the time of the second check.

If you have type 2 diabetes and treat it with healthy eating and exercise only

Check before you eat breakfast. Check 1 or 2 hours after a meal.

DO EXTRA BLOOD GLUCOSE CHECKS

- When your team is trying to find the best dose of insulin or diabetes pills for you
- When you change your exercise program or meal plan
- When you start a new drug that can affect your glucose level
- When you think your glucose is low or high
- When you are sick
- When you are pregnant
- Before and after exercise (during exercise when you have been exercising for more than an hour)
- Before you drive
- Before activities that take a lot of concentration

KEEP RECORDS

Be sure to write down your results, date, and time. Do this even if you have a meter with a memory. Your health care team can tell you what else to record, such as:

- The foods you eat and when you eat them
- Times that you miss meals or snacks
- Times that you eat large or small meals
- Times that you drink alcohol and how much you drink
- How much you weigh
- How much insulin or how many diabetes pills you take and when
- When and how long you exercise
- When and how you treat low or high blood glucose
- When you are ill, injured, stressed, or have just had surgery

Share your records with your health care team. Together, you can make needed changes in your diabetes care plan. A better plan makes it easier for you to care for your diabetes.

Blood Vessel Damage

The enemies of your blood vessels are high blood glucose, high blood pressure, and high blood fats (see Lipids). All four can damage your blood vessels over time. Often, you will not notice any signs until the damage has been done.

When blood vessels are damaged, they become weak, narrow, or blocked. Less blood flows through them to nourish the parts of your body with oxygen. When your body parts get less oxygen, they don't work as well and can become damaged or die. Your heart, brain, or legs and feet might get damaged. Your eyes, kidneys, and nerves might get damaged.

Blood vessel damage comes on slowly. It may begin in childhood and continue throughout life. People with diabetes are more likely to develop blood vessel damage and to get it at a younger age than people without diabetes.

HOW TO REDUCE YOUR RISK OF BLOOD VESSEL DAMAGE

Smoke less or quit. Smoking narrows blood vessels. Quitting can be hard but worth it. You can get support from a stop-smoking program or your health care team.

Control high blood pressure. High blood pressure can weaken blood vessels. Many people can lower their blood pressure by losing weight through healthy eating and exercise. Some people can lower blood pressure by cutting salt intake. Other times, blood pressure drugs are needed. If your doctor has prescribed blood pressure drugs, be sure to take them.

Nudge that cholesterol level down. High cholesterol means more cholesterol in the blood to stick to vessel walls and cause atherosclerosis or hardening of the arteries (see the figure). This is especially true for saturated fats, which are solid at room temperature. These fats include butter, margarine, and lard. Try low-fat or reduced-fat versions of your favorite foods.

Exercise regularly. Even a daily walk around the block helps. Find exercises and activities you enjoy.

Aim for a healthy weight. Being overweight causes your body to leave more fat in your blood. Combine an exercise program with a meal plan that suits your schedule and your tastes.

Get your diabetes under good control. Check your blood glucose. Take your insulin or diabetes pills. Follow your meal plan. Stick with your exercise program. Keep records.

Get regular medical checkups. Your doctor will check for blood vessel damage and help you keep tabs on your blood pressure, blood fat levels, and blood glucose levels.

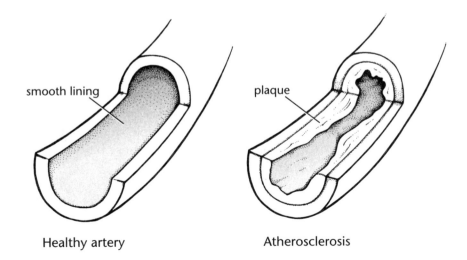

smooth lining

plaque

Healthy artery

Atherosclerosis

Complications

Diabetes can lead to other diseases and conditions called complications. Complications can affect your blood vessels, brain, eyes, heart, kidneys, legs and feet, and nerves.

Your best defenses against complications are keeping your body weight down and your lipid, blood pressure, and blood glucose levels in a normal range. The closer you can get to a normal range, the more likely you are to prevent or delay complications. Both the Diabetes Control and Complications Trial (DCCT) and the United Kingdom Prospective Diabetes Study (UKPDS) proved it.

THE DIABETES CONTROL AND COMPLICATIONS TRIAL

The DCCT was a 10-year-long (1983–1993) medical study sponsored by the National Institutes of Health. It found that people with type 1 diabetes who kept their blood glucose levels close to normal (the level of people without diabetes) had fewer complications than people whose blood glucose levels were higher.

Doctors studied complications in 1,441 people with type 1 diabetes. Some people used a standard therapy for their diabetes. Others used a more intensive therapy.

People on standard therapy injected insulin one or two times each day. Their insulin dose was kept about the same and taken at the same times each day. They checked their urine or blood for glucose. Most people on standard therapy had blood glucose levels above normal. But they did not have really high or low blood glucose levels.

People on intensive therapy injected insulin three or more times a day or used an insulin pump (see Insulin Pumps). They checked their blood glucose four or more times a day. They changed their insulin dose to fit the results of their blood glucose checks, how much they were going to eat, or what exercise they were going to do.

People on intensive therapy had blood glucose levels closer to normal. But they also had severe low blood glucose three times as often and gained more weight than people on the standard therapy.

THE UNITED KINGDOM PROSPECTIVE DIABETES STUDY

The UKPDS is the largest and longest study of people with type 2 diabetes to date. It followed 5,102 people with newly diagnosed type 2 diabetes for an average of 10 years. People were recruited between 1977 and 1991 in 23 centers within the United Kingdom.

Like the DCCT, people were divided into an intensive therapy group and a conventional therapy group. Both groups used various combinations of insulin and/or diabetes pills to lower their blood glucose levels.

The intensive therapy group aimed for a fasting plasma glucose of 108 mg/dl (tight control). The conventional therapy group aimed for a fasting plasma glucose of 270 mg/dl. Those maintaining tight blood glucose control reduced their risk of heart attack, diabetes-related death, eye disease, kidney disease, and possibly nerve disease.

People with high blood pressure were further divided into two groups. Both groups were treated with drugs to lower blood pressure. One group maintained an average blood pressure of 144/82 mmHg (tight control). The other group maintained an average blood pressure of 154/87 mmHg.

People maintaining tight blood pressure control reduced their risk of stroke, diabetes-related death, heart failure, vision loss, and complications of the eyes, kidneys, and nerves.

WHAT THESE STUDIES MEAN FOR YOU

Talk with your diabetes care team about what the results of these studies mean for you. Maybe you want to try for tight control of blood glucose or blood pressure or both. Tight control means keeping your blood glucose and blood pressure levels in a normal range. There is more than one way to gain tight control. You and your diabetes care team can work out a plan for you.

If you keep tight control and still get a complication, it will most likely be milder and slower in coming. If you already have a complication, tight control can keep it from getting worse.

COPING WITH COMPLICATIONS

Learn all you can about your complication. The more you know about your complication, the more in control you will feel.

Talk with family and friends. Tell them what's going on and what they can do to help.

Seek counseling. If you find it hard to talk with family and friends, you may want to get counseling from a social worker or psychologist.

Join a support group. Other people who have your complication can give you moral support. And you may get new ideas on treatment options or doctors. Your health care team or local American Diabetes Association may be able to help you find a support group.

See a specialist. Think about going to a specialist who deals with your complication. Your own doctor may be able to refer you to one.

Ask questions about treatments. What are the treatments? What are the side effects of the treatments? How much do these treatments cost? How often will I need treatments? How many patients with this problem have you treated? What has happened to those patients?

Try to get a second opinion. Check your health insurance. It might cover a second opinion.

Look for organizations that focus on your complication. Organizations such as the National Kidney Foundation, the American Foundation for the Blind, and the National Amputation Foundation have programs and services. To find out more about them, search the Internet or look in *The Encyclopedia of Associations*. It's in most libraries.

Think positive. Thinking good thoughts about yourself and about things in your life can make your life happier. Maybe even longer. Thinking too much about things you don't like or that make you angry or sad can only make living with complications harder for you and your loved ones.

Coping with Diabetes

Diabetes never goes away or even takes a vacation. It is a chronic disease that can be controlled, but not cured. Living with diabetes is not only hard on your body but also hard on your mind.

You may at times deny that you have diabetes or feel angry or depressed about it. These feelings are normal. They may help you cope with having diabetes. They can be part of the process you go through before you accept diabetes.

Accepting diabetes means acknowledging that you have a chronic illness and taking responsibility for managing it, staying in good health, and living a full life. Accepting diabetes means you do not ignore diabetes and let it become a more serious health problem.

The best way to cope with diabetes is to accept it. But what if you get stuck in the process? If you are stuck in denial, anger, or depression for a long time, you may stop taking care of your diabetes.

DENIAL

Almost everybody goes through denial when they are first diagnosed with diabetes. The trouble comes when you keep on denying your diabetes. Continued denial keeps you from learning what you need to know to stay healthy. If you hear yourself thinking or saying some of these words, you may be denying some part of your diabetes care.

"A second helping just this once won't hurt."

"This sore will heal by itself."

"I'll go to the doctor later."

"I don't have time to do it."

"My diabetes isn't serious."

"I only take a pill, not shots."

"I can't because it's not covered by my insurance."

Breaking away from denial

- Write down your diabetes care plan and your health goals. Know why each part of your plan is important. Accept that it will take time to reach your goals.

- Talk to your diabetes educator about your diabetes care plan. Together you may be able to come up with a better plan.

- Tell your friends and family how you take care of your diabetes. Tell them how they can help you.

ANGER

Anger is a powerful emotion. If you don't use anger, it will use you. To gain control over your anger, learn more about it. Start an anger diary. Write down when you felt angry, where you were, who you were with, why you felt angry, and what you did. After a few weeks, read it over. Try to understand your anger. What are you angry about? Usually under your anger are hurt feelings.

The better you understand your anger, the better you will be able to control it. How you use the energy of your anger is up to you. Plan to use your anger in a way that helps you next time.

How to control your anger

Defuse it. Talk slowly, take deep breaths, get a drink of water, sit down, lean back, keep your hands down at your sides.

Let it out. Do a physical activity like jogging or raking leaves. Cry over a sad movie. Write down on a piece of paper what you feel like saying or shouting.

Make it trivial. Ask yourself just how important it is. Some things are just too trivial to be worth your anger.

Laugh at it. Find something funny about it. Sometimes laughter can push out anger.

Let it give you strength. Anger can give you the courage to speak up for yourself or act to protect someone else.

DEPRESSION

Feeling down once in awhile is normal. But feeling really sad and hopeless for 2 weeks or more might be a sign of serious depression.

You may be depressed if

- You no longer take interest or pleasure in things you used to enjoy doing.
- You have trouble falling asleep, wake often during the night, or want to sleep a lot more than usual.
- You wake up earlier than usual and cannot get back to sleep.
- You eat more or less than you used to. You quickly gain or lose weight.
- You have trouble concentrating. Other thoughts or feelings distract you.
- You have no energy. You feel tired all the time.
- You are so nervous or anxious, you can't sit still.
- You are less interested in sex.
- You cry often.
- You feel you never do anything right and are a burden to others.
- You feel sad or worse in the morning than you do the rest of the day.
- You feel you want to die or are thinking about ways to hurt yourself.

If you have three or more of these signs, get help. If you have one or two of these signs and have been feeling bad for 2 weeks or more, get help.

Help for depression

Talk to your doctor first. There may be a physical cause for your depression. If you and your doctor rule out physical causes, your doctor will likely refer you to a mental health professional. Treatment may involve counseling or antidepressant medication or both.

HOW TO COPE WITH DIABETES

Once you have made it through any denial, anger, or depression, you are on your way to accepting your diabetes. Accepting your diabetes is the way to cope with it.

Accept that diabetes care is up to you. You are the one who decides what to eat, how much to exercise, and when to check your blood glucose. Accept this for what it is—control. You are in control.

Learn as much about diabetes as you can. Your local American Diabetes Association can help. Read. Ask questions. Take diabetes education classes. Go to diabetes support groups.

Share what you have learned with your family and friends. The more they know, the better they will be able to help you. Tell them how you feel about diabetes.

Keep active in your hobbies, activities, and sports. You'll show everyone, including yourself, that you're still the same person. You can still have lots of fun.

Dental Care

Having diabetes puts you at risk for gum disease and other mouth infections. Infections can make your blood glucose level go up. And a high blood glucose level can make mouth infections even worse. You can protect yourself by knowing the signs of gum disease and other mouth infections and by knowing how to take care of your teeth.

GUM DISEASE

Gum disease is an infection of your gums. It starts when a sticky film of bacteria, called plaque, forms on your teeth and at your gum line. You need to brush and floss your teeth to remove the plaque, or it hardens into tartar. Plaque and tartar irritate your gums. Your gums can become red, sore, and swollen. Then even gentle brushing can make your gums bleed. This is called gingivitis. If you ignore gingivitis, gum disease can get worse.

As gum disease gets worse, your gums begin to pull away from your teeth. Part of your tooth's root may show or your teeth may look longer. Pockets may form between your teeth and gums. These pockets fill with bacteria and pus. This is called periodontitis.

Periodontitis can destroy your jaw bone. Your teeth may start to move. You may notice a change in the way your teeth fit when you bite or in the way your partial dentures fit. Your teeth may get loose, fall out, or have to be pulled. Know the warning signs of gum disease so you don't let it get this far.

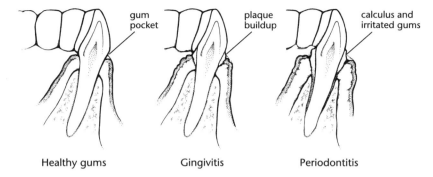

| Healthy gums | Gingivitis | Periodontitis |

gum pocket · plaque buildup · calculus and irritated gums

Signs of gum disease

- Red gums
- Swollen or tender gums
- Gums that bleed when you brush or floss
- Gums that have pulled away from your teeth
- Pus between your teeth and gums when you press on the gums
- Bad breath
- Loose teeth
- Teeth that are moving away from each other
- A change in the way your teeth fit when you bite
- A change in the way your partial dentures fit

See your dentist if you have any of these signs.

OTHER MOUTH INFECTIONS

Mouth infections affect small areas in your mouth rather than your whole mouth. They can be caused by bacteria or a fungus. Know the warning signs of mouth infections.

Signs of mouth infections

- Swelling around your teeth or gums or anywhere in your mouth
- Pus around your teeth or gums or anywhere in your mouth

- White or red patches anywhere in your mouth
- Pain in your mouth or sinuses that does not go away
- Dark spots or holes on your teeth
- Teeth that hurt when you eat something cold, hot, or sweet
- Pain when chewing

See your dentist if you have any of these signs.

HOW TO PROTECT YOUR TEETH

Control your blood glucose. If you keep your blood glucose at healthy levels, you'll lower your risk of gum disease and other mouth infections.

Keep your teeth clean. Brush your teeth with a fluoride toothpaste at least twice a day. Better yet, brush after every meal. Be careful not to brush too hard. You may wear away your gums. A soft toothbrush with rounded or polished bristles is easiest on your gums. Be sure to replace your toothbrush every 3 or 4 months, or sooner if the bristles are worn.

Floss your teeth at least once a day. If you don't like to use floss, try interdental picks or sticks. Flossing or using dental picks cleans plaque and bits of food from between your teeth. Brushing removes plaque and bits of food from the surfaces of your teeth. Another option is an ultrasonic toothbrush, which uses moving bristles and ultrasonic waves to remove plaque between teeth, as well as on the surface.

Go to your dentist. Have your dentist or dental hygienist clean your teeth every 6 months, or more frequently, if necessary. These cleanings get rid of plaque and tartar. Make sure your dentist takes full mouth X-rays every 2 years to check for bone loss. For some people, bone loss is the only sign of periodontitis. Let your dentist know you have diabetes.

Dietitian

A dietitian is an expert in food and nutrition. Food is a key part of your diabetes care. A dietitian can help you figure out your food needs based on your weight, lifestyle, diabetes pills or insulin, other drugs you may be taking, and your health goals. Dietitians can teach you many useful skills, such as how to:

- Make a meal plan
- Use a meal plan
- Fit favorite foods into your meal plan
- Make a sick-day meal plan
- Read food labels
- Choose wisely when grocery shopping
- Choose wisely from restaurant menus
- Turn a fatty recipe into a low-fat one
- Find healthy cookbooks and food guides
- Find out how the foods you eat affect your lipid levels
- Find out how the foods you eat affect your blood glucose levels
- Treat yourself for low blood glucose
- Use your blood glucose records to improve your food choices

When your weight, lifestyle, medical needs, or health goals change, your food needs are likely to change, too. Your dietitian can help you adjust your meal plan to those changes.

The American Diabetes Association recommends that all adults with diabetes see a dietitian every 6 months to a year.

WHEN YOU LOOK FOR A DIETITIAN

Look for the initials RD after a dietitian's name. RD stands for registered dietitian. A registered dietitian has met standards set by The American Dietetic Association. An RD may also have a master's degree.

You might see the initials LD after a dietitian's name. LD stands for licensed dietitian. Many states require dietitians to have a license.

Look for a dietitian who has worked with people who have diabetes. The letters CDE after a dietitian's name mean that he or she is trained and up-to-date in diabetes care and treatment. CDE stands for Certified Diabetes Educator.

Your doctor or local area hospitals may be able to recommend a dietitian. You can also call The American Dietetic Association Consumer Nutrition Hot Line at 1-800-366-1655 or go to *www.eatright.org*.

Doctor

Your diabetes doctor may be an internist, a family practitioner, a general practitioner, a nurse practitioner, or a physician's assistant who cares for people with diabetes. Your doctor may be an endocrinologist or a diabetologist. An endocrinologist is a medical doctor who has special training and certification in treating diseases such as diabetes. A diabetologist is a medical doctor who has a special interest in diabetes.

The kind of diabetes doctor you go to is not as important as the kind of care you get. The American Diabetes Association has guidelines to let your doctor know how to care for you. These guidelines are called "Standards of Medical Care for Patients with Diabetes Mellitus." They can be found in the *Clinical Practice Recommendations,* a yearly supplement to the January issue of the journal *Diabetes Care.* Be sure to let your doctor know about them.

The guidelines can help you, too. They let you know what to expect from your doctor. That way, you can check whether your doctor is giving you the best care. Here's a sample of what the guidelines cover.

FIRST VISIT

During your first visit to a new doctor who will treat your diabetes, ask the doctor to help you put together a health care team (see Health Care Team). At your first visit, your doctor or other health care team member will:

- Ask when you found out you had diabetes
- Ask for results of those lab tests
- Ask who else in your family has diabetes
- Ask how you treat your diabetes
- Ask what and when you eat
- Ask how often and how hard you exercise
- Ask about your weight
- Ask if you smoke
- Ask if you have high blood pressure
- Ask if you have high cholesterol
- Ask if you have had ketones in your urine
- Ask if you have had low blood glucose
- Ask what infections you have had
- Ask what complications you have had
- Ask what treatments you have been given
- Ask what drugs you are taking
- Ask what other medical problems you have had
- Ask if you had problems when pregnant
- Measure your height, weight, and blood pressure
- Look in your eyes and ask about eye problems
- Look in your mouth and ask about dental problems
- Feel your neck to check your thyroid gland and do tests if needed
- Listen to your heart through a stethoscope
- Feel your abdomen to check your liver and other organs
- Look at your hands and fingers
- Look at your bare feet
- Check the sensation and pulses in your feet
- Check your skin
- Test your reflexes
- Take your pulse
- Request blood and urine samples for tests

FUTURE VISITS

Your doctor will tell you when to come for another checkup. Your doctor may want to see you two to four times a year.

If you take insulin or if you are having trouble reaching your blood glucose goals, your doctor may want to see you four or more times a year.

If you have complications or if you start something new in your diabetes care plan, your doctor may want to see you even more often.

When you return, expect your doctor or other health care team members to:

- Ask to see your blood glucose records
- Ask if your blood glucose has been too high or too low
- Ask about signs that might mean you are getting a complication
- Ask if you have been sick since your last visit
- Ask what drugs you are taking now
- Ask if your life has changed
- Ask if you have had problems with your plan
- Weigh you and take your blood pressure
- Look in your eyes
- Look at your bare feet
- Request blood for an A1C test
- Request a urine test
- Request tests of kidney function
- Request tests of blood fat levels
- Go over your plan to see if you have met your goals
- Discuss changes in your plan if you both agree that changes are needed

Eating Disorders

Two eating disorders—anorexia and bulimia—may be more common in people with diabetes. Researchers are not sure why this is so, but both diabetes and eating disorders have in common a focus on food and weight.

ANOREXIA

People with anorexia have an intense fear of becoming fat. To stay thin, they starve themselves. They may have secretive or strange eating habits, such as cutting food into tiny pieces. They may refuse to eat with other people. To lose more weight, they may exercise very hard. People with anorexia see themselves as fat even when they are very thin.

BULIMIA

People with bulimia are overly concerned with their body shape and weight. They will binge and purge twice a week or more to prevent weight gain. Bingeing is eating a large amount of food (often several thousand calories worth) at one time.

During a binge, people with bulimia feel out of control and frightened. After a binge, they feel depressed and have low self-esteem. They purge themselves by making themselves throw up or by taking laxatives or diuretics to cause diarrhea or fluid loss. They may also try to severely control their weight by strict dieting or fasting, or by exercising very hard. People with bulimia may be overweight, underweight, or of normal weight.

EATING DISORDERS AND DIABETES CONTROL

Most people with diabetes who have an eating disorder have poor diabetes control. A few manage to keep their diabetes in good control. Those with bulimia may take more insulin after a binge. Those with anorexia may lower their insulin dose to match their lower food intake. Others just work hard to keep their eating disorder under control so that they do not upset their diabetes control.

EATING DISORDERS AND WEIGHT CONTROL

An eating disorder makes weight control very difficult. People with diabetes who have an eating disorder may reduce or omit their insulin dose to lose weight. Many people who try this are overweight. Others are of normal weight or even low weight.

Stopping insulin causes a dangerous kind of weight loss. The body loses water weight and can become dehydrated. Without enough insulin, the body does not get enough blood glucose for energy. The body uses up its stores of glycogen in the liver. Then it starts to break down fat tissues, muscles, and body organs. If insulin is not resumed, the person eventually dies.

EATING DISORDERS AND HEALTH

People with eating disorders are more likely to have digestion problems, heart problems, and other problems brought on by starvation, self-induced vomiting, and abuse of laxatives and diuretics. In addition, people with diabetes who have an eating disorder are more likely to get:

- High ketones
- High blood glucose
- Low blood glucose
- Eye disease
- Kidney disease
- Nerve disease

HELP FOR EATING DISORDERS

A person with an eating disorder needs the help of a physician, mental health professional, and dietitian. Ask a family doctor or counselor for a referral. Some clinics and health care centers specialize in treating people with eating disorders. Check the white pages of a phone book under "Eating Disorders." You might also be able to find information or a support group through the Internet.

Most eating disorders can be treated with outpatient psychotherapy or behavioral therapy and family or group therapy. Drugs for depression are sometimes used. If a person with an eating disorder refuses help and his or her life is in danger, he or she may be admitted to the psychiatric unit of a hospital for treatment.

Employment Rights

Some employers are afraid to hire people who have diabetes. They worry that diabetes will interfere with the job. Or that it will make health insurance premiums higher for the company. Because of this, people who have diabetes may have a harder time finding jobs than people who do not have diabetes. And they may lose jobs more easily. As a worker with diabetes, you should be aware of your legal rights and how to protect those rights.

ANTIDISCRIMINATION LAWS

Several federal laws prohibit discrimination in the workplace based on disability. The Americans with Disabilities Act applies to private employers, labor unions, employment agencies with 1 or more employees, and state and local government. The Rehabilitation Act of 1973 generally covers employees who work for the executive branch of the federal government or for an employer that receives federal money. The Congressional Accountability Act covers employees of Congress and most legislative branch agencies.

These laws prohibit an employer from taking any adverse employment action because of a person's disability. This means that an employer cannot discriminate in hiring, firing, discipline, pay, promotion, job training, fringe benefits, or any other term or condition of employment. Employers are also prohibited from retaliating against an employee for asserting his or her rights. You are usually not required to tell employers that you have diabetes, but the laws protect you from discrimination only if your employer knows about your disability.

In order to be protected by these antidiscrimination laws, you must show that you are a "qualified individual with a disability." The first step is establishing that you have a disability. A disability is defined in these laws as a mental or physical impairment that substantially limits one or more major life activities—such as walking, seeing, or working. If you have a previous record of a disability, this can be used to establish your disability now.

You also have to establish that you are qualified for the job in question. You are considered a qualified worker if you satisfy the skill, experience, education, and other job-related requirements of the position held or desired, and—if you're given reasonable accommodation—you can perform the essential functions of that position. An accommodation is any change or adjustment to a job or work environment that enables you to do the job.

All states have their own antidiscrimination laws and agencies responsible for enforcing these laws.

In addition, the Family and Medical Leave Act requires most private employers with over 50 employees, and most government employers, to provide up to 12 weeks of leave per year because of a worker's, or an immediate family member's, serious health condition.

ACCOMMODATIONS

As stated above, employers are required to make a "reasonable accommodation" if requested by an employee with a disability, unless the accommodation would cause an "undue hardship" on the employer because of significant difficulty or expense. The accommodations that people with diabetes need are usually easy and inexpensive. For example, you might require accommodations such as:

- Breaks to check blood glucose levels, eat a snack, or go to the bathroom
- The ability to keep diabetes supplies and food nearby
- The opportunity to work a modified schedule or to work a standard shift, as opposed to a swing shift.

ADDRESSING DISCRIMINATION

Educate and negotiate. Discrimination based on diabetes is often the result of ignorance. Problems can sometimes be resolved by educating others about the disease and about your medical needs and abilities. When education alone is not enough, try to figure out a compromise that benefits everyone.

Litigate. Sometimes it takes legal action to end discrimination. Usually, you are required to begin by filing a charge of discrimination with the appropriate government agency. If the employer is a private company or state or local government, file a charge with either the Equal Employment Opportunity Commission or your state antidiscrimination agency. If the employer is the federal government, contact the internal Equal Employment Opportunity office of the agency where the discrimination occurred. You must act promptly because the time limits for taking action are often very short. If the agency does not resolve the problem to your satisfaction, you can file a lawsuit in federal or state court claiming discrimination on the basis of disability.

Legislate. Sometimes it is necessary to work to change laws and policies that are unfair to people with diabetes.

If you want more information about employment rights, call 1-800-DIABETES for the ADA's packet on employment discrimination or to discuss a specific employment problem with ADA's Legal Advocate.

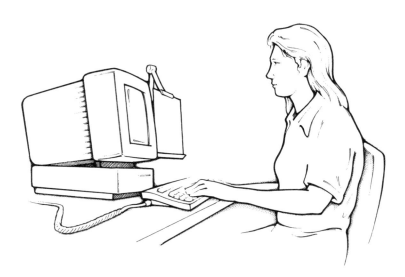

Exercise, Aerobic

Aerobic exercises are ones that use your heart, lungs, arms, and legs. By working these parts of your body, you can improve your blood flow, reduce your risk of heart disease, and lower your blood pressure. You can also lower your LDL cholesterol and triglycerides and raise your HDL cholesterol (the good kind).

When you do aerobic exercises, you breathe harder and your heart beats faster. This builds your endurance and increases your energy. You may find that aerobic exercise helps you sleep better, makes you feel less stressed, balances your emotions, and improves your sense of well-being.

Aerobic exercise is not only good for your health but is also good for your diabetes. Aerobic exercise helps your insulin to work more efficiently, reduces your body fat, and helps you lose weight. If you don't exercise already, your doctor may advise you to start.

WHAT TO DO BEFORE YOU START

Check with your doctor before you start any exercise. Your doctor may want to run some tests to see how your heart, blood vessels, eyes, feet, and nerves are doing. Your blood pressure, blood fat levels, A1C levels, and body fat might also be checked. Your health care team can help you learn how to adjust your diabetes care plan for exercise.

WHAT AEROBIC EXERCISES TO DO

Some exercises may make heart, eye, feet, or nerve problems worse. Find out from your doctor or an exercise physiologist what kinds of exercises are safe for you to do. Pick from these exercises a few you think you might enjoy. Then learn the right way to do each exercise.

Examples of aerobic exercises

- Aerobics classes or videotapes
- Bicycling
- Dancing
- Jogging
- Jumping rope
- Rowing
- Running
- Skating (roller, ice, in-line)
- Skiing (downhill, cross-country)
- Stair climbing
- Swimming
- Walking
- Water exercises

HOW LONG AND HOW OFTEN TO EXERCISE

If you are just starting to exercise after a long time of little or no activity, go for 5 minutes. Build up to short bouts of exercise that add up to at least 30 minutes a day. For example, you might try brisk walking or stair climbing for 10 minutes three times a day or for 15 minutes twice a day.

Exercising for less than 15 minutes a day is not likely to improve your health. Gradually build up to 20 to 60 minutes of continuous aerobic exercise three to five times a week. The 20 to 60 minutes of aerobic exercise does not include your warm-up and cooldown.

A warm-up will slowly raise your heart rate, warm your muscles, and help prevent injuries. A cooldown will lower your heart rate and slow your breathing. Warm up for 5 to 10 minutes before aerobic exercise, and cool down for 5 to 10 minutes after aerobic exercise. As a warm-up or a cooldown, you could gently stretch, walk, or slowly bicycle.

HOW HARD TO EXERCISE

Your doctor or exercise specialist can tell you how hard to exercise by giving you a pulse count number. The number is a percentage of your maximum heart rate, which indicates your capacity for exercise. It may be as low as 55% or as high as 79%. Here's one easy way to figure out your pulse count.

Calculating your target zone

- Subtract your age from 220 to figure out your maximal heart rate (HRmax).

  (Example for someone 40 years old)

  220 − your age = HRmax

  220 − 40 years old = 180

- Multiply your HRmax by 55% and 79% to figure out your target zone in heartbeats per minute (or 55% and 65% if you are just starting out).

  HRmax × 0.55 = bottom of your target zone   180 × 0.55 = 108
  HRmax × 0.79 = top of your target zone   180 × 0.79 = 144

- Divide your target zone numbers (heart-beats per minute) by 6 to figure out your 10-second pulse count.

  Bottom target ÷ 6 = Bottom 10-second count   108 ÷ 6 = 18
  Top target ÷ 6 = Top 10-second count   144 ÷ 6 = 24

So, using this easy formula, we can see that a 40-year-old man would have a target zone of between 18 and 24 heartbeats every 10 seconds.

If you have nerve damage or take certain blood pressure drugs, your heart may beat more slowly. Check with your doctor about this. If your heart does beat more slowly, your heart rate is not a good guide for how hard to exercise. Instead, exercise at what you feel is a moderate level of exertion. Moderate is not too hard and not too easy. You should be able to talk while you're exercising.

Signs that you are exercising too hard

- You can't talk while exercising.
- Your pulse is higher than the pulse you are trying to maintain.
- You rate your level of exertion as hard or very hard.

WHEN TO CHECK YOUR BLOOD GLUCOSE

Exercise usually makes your blood glucose level go down. But if your blood glucose level is high before you start, exercise can make it go up even higher.

If you take insulin or certain diabetes pills (the sulfonylureas, the meglitinides), exercise can make your blood glucose level go too low. The best way to find out how exercise affects your blood glucose is to check before and after exercising.

Check your blood glucose twice before exercise. Check at 30 minutes before exercise and again just before you begin. This tells you whether your blood glucose level is rising, stable, or dropping. If it is higher than 250–300 mg/dl and rising, wait until it is stable. If it is dropping rapidly and below 100 mg/dl, you may need an extra snack to get it stable. When it is stable, begin your exercise.

Be ready to check your blood glucose during exercise. There are times during exercise that you may want to stop and check your blood glucose, such as:

- When you are trying an exercise for the first time and want to see how it is affecting your blood glucose
- When you feel your blood glucose might be going too low
- When you will be exercising for more than 1 hour (check every 30 minutes)

Check your blood glucose after exercise. When you exercise, your body uses glucose that is stored in your muscles and liver. After exercise, your body restores glucose to your muscles and liver by removing it from your blood. This can go on for as long as 10 to 24 hours. During this time, blood glucose levels may fall too low.

WHEN TO EAT SNACKS

Depending on how hard and how long you exercise, you may need to eat extra snacks. A snack can be 1 carbohydrate choice, which provides 15 grams of carb, such as a piece of fruit, half a cup of juice, half a bagel, or a small roll. Talk with your dietitian about what snacks are good for you and when it is best for you to eat them. If you take insulin or certain diabetes pills (the sulfonylureas, the meglitinides), you may need to eat a snack before, during, or after exercise.

If your blood glucose level is less than 100 mg/dl before exercise

You may need to eat a snack before you start.

If your blood glucose level is between 100 and 150 mg/dl before exercise AND you will be exercising for more than 1 hour

You will need to eat 15 grams of carbohydrate every 30 minutes to 1 hour.

If your blood glucose level is between 100 and 250 mg/dl before exercise AND you will be exercising for less than 1 hour

You probably will not need to eat a snack before you start.

If your blood glucose level is below 100 mg/dl during exercise

You may need to eat a snack during exercise.

If your blood glucose level is below 100 mg/dl after exercise

You may need to eat a snack after exercise.

WHEN AND WHAT TO DRINK

Exercise makes you sweat. Sweating means you are losing fluid. To replace lost fluids, be sure to drink after exercise or during exercise if the exercise is intense.

Water is usually the best choice. But if you are exercising for a long time, you may want a drink that contains carbohydrate. Choose drinks that are no more than 10 percent carbohydrate, such as sports drinks or diluted fruit juices (1/2 cup fruit juice, 1/2 cup water).

WHEN TO EXERCISE

A good time to exercise is 1 to 3 hours after you finish a meal or snack. The food you have eaten will help keep your blood glucose level from falling too low. This may not be true if you are using rapid-acting insulin. In this case, talk with your health care team about the appropriate time to exercise.

WHEN NOT TO EXERCISE

- Your blood glucose level stays over 300 mg/dl.
- Your insulin or diabetes pills are peaking.
- You have ketones in your urine.
- You have numbness, tingling, or pain in your feet or legs.
- You are short of breath.
- You are ill.
- You have a serious injury.
- You feel dizzy.
- You feel sick to your stomach.
- You have pain/tightness in your chest, neck, shoulders, or jaw.
- You have blurred sight or blind spots.

Report any unusual symptoms to your health care team.

Exercise, Flexibility

Flexibility is how far you can stretch your muscles around your joints without stiffness, resistance, or pain. Flexible muscles and joints are less likely to get injured when you use them.

One of the best ways to become more flexible is to stretch every day. Stretch a little bit throughout the day to relieve muscle tension and stress. Make stretching a part of your workout.

There are lots of different stretches. You can find them in books, on videos, and in exercise classes. Here are a few stretches for you to try. But first, some rules.

STRETCHING RULES

- Go slowly and smoothly.
- Remember to breathe.
- Don't bounce.
- Relax and let go of any tension you feel.
- Go only as far as you can without pain.
- Hold for at least 10–20 seconds.

Calf stretch. Face a wall and stand about a foot away. Stand with one foot in front of the other, toes straight ahead. Keep both feet flat on the floor. Bend your front knee. Slowly lean forward and rest your forearms on the wall. Press your rear heel into the floor. Repeat with your other leg.

Quadriceps (front of thigh) stretch. Stand with legs slightly bent. Bend one leg back, lifting your foot off the floor. Grab the ankle of the bent leg with one hand. You may want to hold on to something for balance. Gently pull your foot up so your heel is headed for your bottom and hold. Release. Repeat with your other leg.

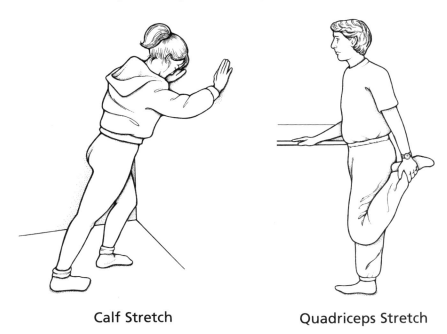

Calf Stretch   Quadriceps Stretch

Hamstrings (back of thigh) stretch. Lie on your back. Bend your legs, feet on the floor. Lift one leg up. Keep it slightly bent. Grasp the leg at the thigh just above the knee with both hands. Holding on to your leg, try to straighten it. Release. Straighten again and release. Repeat with your other leg.

Back and hips stretch. Sit with one leg straight out. Bend your other leg. Cross your bent leg over your straight leg, placing the foot of your bent leg on the floor next to the knee of the straight leg. Breathe. Slowly twist your upper body in the direction of your straight leg. Keep turning your head to look behind you. Keep your shoulders relaxed and your chin level. Brace yourself by placing the elbow of the arm nearest your bent knee on the inside of your bent knee. Slowly unwind and rest both legs on the floor. Repeat on the other side.

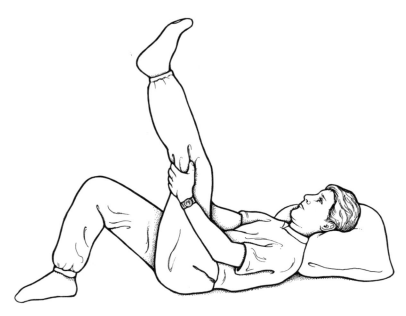

Hamstrings (back of thigh) Stretch

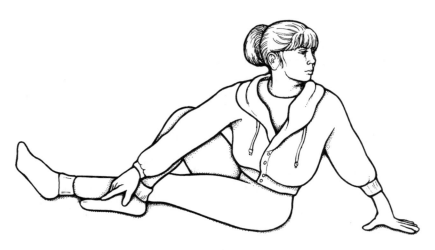

Back and Hips Stretch

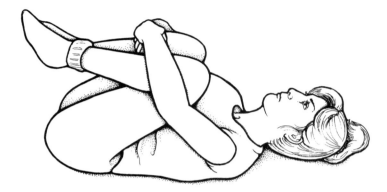

Lower Back Stretch

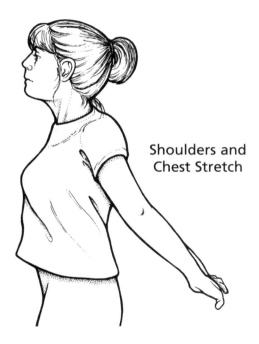

Shoulders and
Chest Stretch

Lower back stretch. Lie on your back. Bring your knees to your chest. Hold your knees with your arms. Hug your knees to your chest and press your lower back into the floor. Release arms. Lower legs.

Shoulders and chest stretch. Lace your fingers together behind you. Lift your arms up. Hold. Breathe. Slowly lower and let go.

Arms stretch. Raise your arms over your head. Lace your fingers together with palms up. Press your arms upward.

Neck stretch. Center your head over your shoulders. Look down. Let your head roll toward your chest. Bring your head back to the center. Look over one shoulder. Bring your head back to the center. Look over the other shoulder. Repeat slowly.

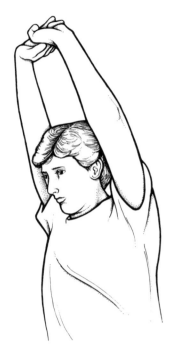

Arms Stretch

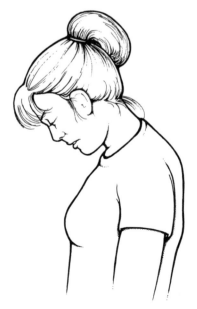

Neck Stretch 1

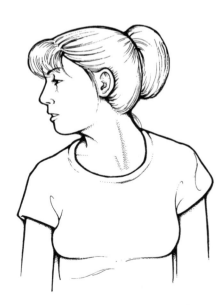

Neck Stretch 2

If you would like more of a challenge for your muscles and joints, consider one of these other forms of exercise that promote flexibility:

- Ballet
- Pilates
- Martial arts
- Modern dance
- Yoga (See Yoga)
- Water aerobics

Before you try any of these flexibility exercises, check with your doctor. Some of the movements may not be safe for you.

You can best learn these flexibility exercises from an instructor. Many places offer classes for beginners. Community recreation centers often have classes at low cost.

If you are thinking of taking a class, you may want to watch at least one class before signing up. You might also want to ask whether the teacher has experience teaching people with diabetes.

Exercise, Strength

Strength exercises are ones that work your muscles against a weight. Strength exercises include using weight machines, exercise bands, medicine balls, or stability balls; lifting free weights; doing calisthenics; or circuit training.

WEIGHT MACHINES

Weight machines allow you to change how much weight you want to lift by either placing a pin in a stack of weights or turning a valve that controls fluid pressure. Some well-known brands of weight machines are Nautilus, Universal, and Cybex.

FREE WEIGHTS

Free weights are not attached to another piece of equipment. Free weights include dumbbells and barbells. A dumbbell is a short bar you can lift with one hand. A barbell is a long bar you lift with both hands.

CALISTHENICS

In calisthenics, the weight you use is your own body. Calisthenics include push-ups, pull-ups, sit-ups, leg lifts, and squats. You can make your muscles work harder by strapping weights to your wrists or ankles or by using elastic bands.

CIRCUIT TRAINING

In circuit training, you go through a series of stations. At each station, you do a different exercise. You might use a weight machine, lift free weights, do an aerobic exercise, or do calisthenics. After you finish the exercise at one station, you have a short rest period before you go on to the next station.

WHY DO STRENGTH EXERCISES?

Strength exercises make your muscles stronger and more flexible and your bones sturdier. Strong muscles and bones are less likely to become injured. The stronger you are, the easier everyday physical tasks become, and the longer you can stay active without tiring.

WHAT TO DO BEFORE YOU START

See your doctor. Talk to your doctor before you start strength exercises. Some exercises may be better for you than others. Some may not be safe for you at all.

Choose your exercises. When you know the kinds of strength exercises that are safe for you, pick out 8 to 10 different ones. Be sure to pick ones that will work your legs and hips, chest, back, shoulders, arms, and abdomen. The idea is to work all your muscle groups. Your health care team may be able to help you choose these exercises.

Learn how to do your exercises. Once you have chosen your exercises, learn the right way to do them. If you do exercises the wrong way, you might injure yourself. If the exercises you have chosen require you to use equipment that is new to you, learn how to use and adjust it. Find out how to use any safety equipment that goes along with your exercise, too.

HOW TO STRENGTHEN WITH WEIGHTS OR CALISTHENICS

As with any other exercise, warm up for 5 to 10 minutes before you begin, and cool down for 5 to 10 minutes after you finish. Try gentle stretching and slow walking or bicycling.

After you warm up, start with just 1 set of each exercise. A set is the number of times you repeat an exercise before you rest. Have an exercise specialist help you figure out how many repetitions to do of each exercise. Here are some general guidelines:

If the strength exercise is easy for you

Do it 15 to 20 times. Rest for 1 minute or less between sets.

If the strength exercise is moderate for you

Do it 8 to 12 times. Rest for 1 or 2 minutes between sets.

If the strength exercise is hard for you

Do it 2 to 6 times. Rest for 3 to 5 minutes between sets.

Remember, start with just 1 set. As you become stronger, you will be able to do more sets. Work your way up a little bit at a time to 2 or 3 sets of each exercise. Once you are doing 2 or 3 sets easily, you are ready to make the exercise harder by adding more weight.

Another thing to remember is to move your muscles through their full range of motion. This increases flexibility. A muscle that moves only part of the way loses flexibility. And keep breathing! Breathe in as you lower. Breathe out as you lift. If you don't like this pattern, then just breathe normally.

HOW LONG AND HOW OFTEN TO EXERCISE

Do your strength exercises for 20 to 30 minutes two or three times a week. Allow at least 1 day of rest between days you do the same strength exercises. To grow stronger, muscles need rest as well as exercise.

Eye Diseases

People with diabetes are more likely to get an eye disease than people without diabetes. The three main eye diseases that people with diabetes get are retinopathy, cataracts, and glaucoma. Of the three, retinopathy is the most common.

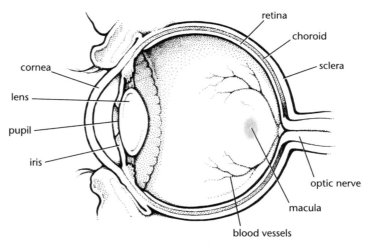

Cross-section of the eye

RETINOPATHY

The retina is the lining at the back of the eye that senses light. Small blood vessels bring oxygen to the retina. Retinopathy damages the small blood vessels in the retina. The two major types of retinopathy are called nonproliferative and proliferative.

Nonproliferative retinopathy

In nonproliferative retinopathy, the small blood vessels in the retina bulge and form pouches. This weakens the blood vessels. They may leak a bit of fluid. This leaking does not usually harm your sight. And often, the disease never gets worse.

If the disease does get worse, the weak blood vessels leak a larger amount of fluid. They also leak blood and fats. This causes the retina to swell. The swelling will usually not harm your sight, unless it occurs in the center of the retina.

The center of the retina is called the macula. The macula lets you see fine details. Swelling in the macula is called macular edema. Macular edema can blur, distort, reduce, or darken your sight.

Proliferative retinopathy

Nonproliferative retinopathy may progress to proliferative retinopathy. In proliferative retinopathy, the small blood vessels are so damaged that they close off. In response, many new blood vessels grow in the retina. As these new blood vessels grow, they branch out to other parts of your eye.

These changes may not affect your sight. Or, these changes will make you less able to see things out of the sides of your eyes. You might also find it harder to see in the dark and to adjust from light to dark.

The new blood vessels are weak and can cause problems. They may break and bleed into the clear gel that fills the center of the eye. This is known as a vitreous hemorrhage. The most common signs of vitreous hemorrhage are blurring and floating spots. Vitreous hemorrhage can cause you to lose sight if not treated.

The new blood vessels may cause scar tissue to grow on the retina. Scar tissue can wrinkle the retina and pull it out of place. A retina that has been pulled away from the back of the eye is called a detached retina. A detached retina will cause you to see a shadow or large dark area. It can endanger your sight.

Signs of retinopathy

- Your sight gets blurry.
- You see floating spots.

- You see a shadow or dark area.
- You can't see things out of the sides of your eyes.
- You have trouble seeing at night.
- You have trouble reading.
- Straight lines do not look straight.

If you have any of these signs, go to your eye doctor right away.

Special note: Usually, you can't see (or feel) the early signs of damage to your retina, but your eye doctor can. Be sure to have your eyes checked for retinopathy every year.

CATARACTS

A cataract clouds the eye's lens. The eye's lens is usually clear. The lens lies behind the iris (the colored part of your eye) and the pupil (the dark opening). The lens focuses light onto the retina. Clouding of the lens blocks light from entering.

Cataracts usually start out small. Some of them never worsen your sight. Others block most or all of your sight. How a cataract will affect your sight depends on three things: 1) how large or small it is, 2) how thin or thick it is, and 3) where it is on the lens.

Because of these three things, signs that you have a cataract may vary.

Signs of a cataract

- Your sight is hazy, fuzzy, or blurry.
- You think you need new glasses.
- Your new glasses don't help you see any better.
- You find it harder to read and do other close work.
- You blink a lot to see better.
- You feel you have a film over your eyes.
- You feel you are looking through a cloudy piece of glass, veils, or a waterfall.

- Light from the sun or a lamp seems too bright.
- At night, headlights on other cars cause more glare than before or look double or dazzling.
- Your pupil, which is usually black, looks gray, yellow, or white.
- Colors look dull.

If you have any of these signs, see your eye doctor.

GLAUCOMA

Glaucoma is a buildup of fluid in the eye. The fluid buildup causes increased pressure. The pressure can damage your optic nerve. Your optic nerve tells your brain what your eye sees. There are two kinds of glaucoma.

The most common type is chronic open-angle glaucoma. In this type, fluid pressure rises slowly over many years. You usually won't notice it. You might feel the increased pressure in your eye or your eyes may keep tearing.

As the glaucoma worsens, you may notice that your sight is slightly blurry or foggy. You may feel that your glasses should be changed. You may have a hard time seeing in the dark. If not treated, you may lose your sight.

The less common type of glaucoma is acute angle-closure glaucoma. In this type, fluid pressure builds up quickly. Your eyes hurt a lot. They are blurry and keep tearing. You see colored halos around bright lights. You may even vomit. *If you have any of these signs, go to a hospital emergency room right away.*

HOW TO KEEP YOUR EYES FREE OF DISEASE

Keep your blood glucose levels close to normal. Keeping your blood glucose levels close to normal lowers your risk of getting eye diseases and slows down those that have started.

Control high blood pressure. High blood pressure can make eye diseases worse. You may be able to bring blood pressure down by losing weight, eating less salt, and avoiding alcohol. Your doctor can tell you about drugs to lower blood pressure.

Quit smoking. Smoking damages your blood vessels.

Lower high cholesterol. High cholesterol can also damage your blood vessels.

Get yearly dilated eye and visual exams by an eye doctor. Many eye diseases can do damage without causing signs you can see. An eye doctor has the tools and tests to find damage early. The earlier damage is found, the greater the chance that treatments can save your sight.

Food Labeling

Food labels tell you almost everything you need to know about the foods you buy. The more you know about foods, the better food choices you can make, and the better you can follow your healthy eating plan (see Healthy Eating; and Meal Planning).

One of the first things you might see on a food package is a nutrient claim, such as "reduced fat" or "low calorie." These claims have standard meanings. Some of these terms and their meanings are listed at the end of this section. But the most useful information on a food package is found in the Nutrition Facts box.

SERVING SIZES

Serving sizes are now more uniform in all brands of similar foods. In this way, you can more easily make comparisons. And the serving sizes are closer to the amounts people really eat. Serving sizes are given in both household (e.g., cup) and metric (e.g., gram) measures. The label also gives the number of servings per container.

LIST OF NUTRIENTS

Nutrition Facts list calories, calories from fat, total fat, saturated fat, cholesterol, sodium, total carbohydrate, fiber, sugars, and protein. Nutrients that may also be listed include calories from saturated fat, polyunsaturated fat, and monounsaturated fat. Nutrients listed are followed by a number. This number is the amount of that nutrient in grams (g) or milligrams (mg) in one serving of the food.

Nutrition Facts

Serving Size 1 cup (228g)
Servings Per Container 2

Amount Per Serving

Calories 260   Calories from Fat 120

	% Daily Value*
Total Fat 13g	**20%**
Saturated Fat 5g	**25%**
Cholesterol 30mg	**10%**
Sodium 660mg	**28%**
Total Carbohydrate 31g	**10%**
Dietary Fiber 0g	**0%**
Sugars 5g	
Protein 5g	

Vitamin A 4%	•	Vitamin C 2%
Calcium 15%	•	Iron 4%

* Percent Daily Values are based on a 2,000 calorie diet. Your daily values may be higher or lower depending on your calorie needs:

	Calories:	2,000	2,500
Total Fat	Less than	65g	80g
Sat Fat	Less than	20g	25g
Cholesterol	Less than	300mg	300mg
Sodium	Less than	2,400mg	2,400mg
Total Carbohydrate		300g	375g
Dietary Fiber		25g	30g

Calories per gram:
Fat 9 • Carbohydrate 4 • Protein 4

BASIC FOOD LABEL
Source: Food and Drug Administration

VITAMINS AND MINERALS

Nutrition Facts also list the amounts of vitamin A, vitamin C, calcium, and iron. Other vitamins and minerals may be listed. After the name of the vitamin or mineral is a number followed by a percent sign (%). This number is the percentage of the daily amount of the vitamin or mineral in one serving of the food. Higher numbers mean the food has more of that vitamin or mineral.

DAILY VALUES

Daily Values tell you how much total fat, saturated fat, cholesterol, sodium, potassium, total carbohydrate, fiber, and protein you need each day based on the number of calories you eat in a day. There is no Daily Value for sugars.

All Nutrition Facts labels give Daily Values for a person eating 2,000 calories a day. Some labels also list Daily Values for a person eating 2,500 calories a day.

Your own Daily Values may be higher or lower than those on the label. The more calories you need to eat in a day, the higher your Daily Values. The fewer calories you need to eat in a day, the lower your Daily Values. With the help of a dietitian, you can figure out your own Daily Values to fit your calorie needs.

Percent Daily Values

Percent (%) Daily Values, listed on the right side of the Nutrition Facts label, tell you what percentage of the Daily Value you are getting in one serving of the food.

INGREDIENTS LIST

Ingredients are listed on food packages according to their weight. The ingredient weighing the most is listed first. The ingredient listed last weighs the least. It pays to read the ingredients list, because claims on packages can be misleading.

USING FOOD LABELS

The Nutrition Facts on a food label will tell you exactly how many grams of carbohydrate, grams of fat, and calories are in a serving of food. This makes carbohydrate counting, fat gram counting, and calorie counting straightforward.

If you use the *Exchange Lists for Meal Planning* (see Meal Planning), you will need to compare the serving size on the label to the serving size of an exchange. They may not be the same. For example, the label may list a serving size as 1 cup, but the exchange may list the serving size as 1/2 cup. In this case, 1 cup of the food would be equal to 2 exchanges.

NUTRIENT CLAIMS

Term	Description
Calorie free	Less than 5 calories per serving
Cholesterol free	Less than 2 mg of cholesterol per serving and 2 g or less of saturated fat per serving
Fat free	Less than 0.5 g of fat per serving
Saturated fat free	Less than 0.5 g of saturated fat per serving
Sodium free	Less than 5 mg of sodium per serving
Sugar free	Less than 0.5 g of sugar per serving
Low calorie	40 calories or less per serving
Low cholesterol	20 mg or less of cholesterol per serving and 2 g or less of saturated fat per serving
Low fat	3 g or less of fat per serving
Low saturated fat	1 g or less of saturated fat per serving
Low sodium	140 mg or less of sodium per serving
Extra lean	Less than 5 g of fat, 2 g of saturated fat, and 95 mg of cholesterol per serving
Lean	Less than 10 g of fat, 4.5 g of saturated fat, and 95 mg of cholesterol per serving
Light or lite	33.3% fewer calories or 50% less fat per serving than comparison food
Reduced	25% less per serving than comparison food. Check label carefully. Some of these foods are still too high in fat and calories.

Foot Care

People with diabetes can get many kinds of foot problems. Even minor ones can turn into serious ones.

NERVE DAMAGE

Nerve damage can make your feet less able to feel pain, heat, and cold. Nerve damage can affect the nerves that cause sweating. As a result of decreased sweating, your feet may become dry and scaly. The skin may peel and crack. Nerve damage can also deform your feet. Your toes may curl up. The ball of your foot may stick out more. Your arch may get higher. These changes can cause some parts of your feet to bear more weight. Those areas are then more likely to get corns and calluses (see below).

If you have lost some of the feeling in your feet

- Don't go barefoot. You could hurt your foot and not notice it. If you are going swimming or wading, wear footwear made for water.
- Check your shoes before putting them on. Make sure there are no stones, nails, paper clips, pins, or other sharp objects in them. Be sure the inside of the shoe is smooth and free of tears or rough edges.

If your feet sweat a lot

- Try wearing socks made of silk or thin polypropylene under your regular socks. They wick away sweat and help reduce friction. Be sure you have enough room in your shoes to fit both pairs of socks. You can also buy specialty socks that are designed to wick away sweat. These socks are available at most athletic stores.

If your feet are dry and scaly

- Use a moisturizer twice a day. But don't put the moisturizer between your toes. The extra moisture can lead to infection.
- Don't soak your feet. Soaking dries out your skin.

If the shape of your foot has changed

- Ask your diabetes care provider or foot doctor about shoe inserts or special shoes.

CORNS AND CALLUSES

Calluses are areas of thick skin caused by regular or prolonged pressure or friction. A corn is a callus on a toe. Corns and calluses can develop on your feet when your body weight is borne unevenly. There are several things you can do to prevent calluses from forming.

Wear shoes that fit. Shoes that fit are comfortable when you buy them. Almost all new shoes are a little stiff at the start and mold to your feet with wear. But this is different from buying the wrong size and trying to break them in. Make sure there is room for you to move your toes.

Wear shoes with low heels and thick soles. Thick soles will cushion and protect your feet. Low heels distribute your weight more evenly.

Try padded socks. They not only cushion and protect feet but also reduce pressure. Be sure your shoe is large enough to fit this thicker sock. You may need extra-deep shoes.

Try shoe inserts. Ask your diabetes care provider or foot doctor about shoe inserts to better distribute your weight onto your feet.

If you get a callus or corn, have it trimmed by your diabetes doctor or foot doctor. Trying to cut corns or calluses yourself can lead to infections. Trying to remove them with over-the-counter chemicals can burn your skin. Untrimmed calluses can get very thick, break down, and turn into ulcers.

FOOT ULCERS

Foot ulcers are open sores or holes in the skin. Ulcers form most often over the ball of the foot or on the bottom of the big toe. They can also form on the sole, the heel, or the other toes. Ulcers can be caused by a cut, callus, or blister that is not taken care of. Ulcers on the sides of a foot are usually caused by shoes that don't fit well. You can prevent ulcers by:

- Wearing shoes that fit
- Wearing new shoes for just a few hours at a time
- Throwing away worn-out shoes and sneakers
- Wearing socks that fit
- Wearing socks without seams, holes, or bumpy areas in them
- Putting on clean socks each day
- Putting or rolling your socks on gently
- Checking for pebbles or other objects before you put your shoes on

An ulcer can be very painful. But if you have nerve damage (see above), you may not feel it. Even though you may not feel any pain from an ulcer, you need to get medical attention right away. Walking on an ulcer can cause it to become larger and infected. An infected ulcer can lead to gangrene and amputation (see below).

POOR CIRCULATION

Damage to the blood vessels in the legs and feet can lead to poor circulation. Poor circulation can make your feet feel cold or look blue or swollen.

If your feet are cold

- Wear warm socks.
- Do not use hot water bottles, heating pads, or electric blankets. They may burn your feet without your noticing.
- Keep your feet out of water that is too hot or too cold. Check the water first with your elbow.

If your feet are swollen

- Try shoes that lace up. You can tighten or loosen the laces to fit the shoes to the shape of your feet.

Poor circulation can slow the healing of wounds and infections. It can also cause dry gangrene (see below). Be alert to the signs of blood vessel damage to the legs and feet.

Signs of blood vessel damage to the legs and feet

- Cramping or tightness in one or both legs while walking but not at rest, known as intermittent claudication
- Cold feet
- Pain in the legs or feet while at rest
- Loss of hair on the feet
- Shiny skin
- Thickened toenails

GANGRENE AND AMPUTATION

Gangrene is death of tissues. There are two types of gangrene: dry and wet. Dry gangrene can be treated by improving blood circulation to the foot. Antibiotics can be taken to prevent the area from becoming infected with bacteria. If infection sets in, you have wet gangrene. The only treatment for wet gangrene is amputation. Amputation is removal of the dead tissues. It might mean you lose a toe, several toes, a foot, or part of a foot.

Special note: Almost all people with diabetes who need amputations are smokers.

HOW TO CARE FOR YOUR FEET

Check both your feet each day. Look all over your feet. If you cannot see well, have a friend or relative who can see well do it for you. Compare one foot to the other. Use a mirror to help see the bottom of your feet. Look for any of these foot problems:

Cuts	Blisters
Cracks	Breaks
Scratches	Calluses
Ingrown toenails	Swelling
Redness	Changes in color
Changes in shape	Pain
Cold spots	Loss of feeling
Hot spots	Corns
Ulcers	Dryness
Holes	Peeling

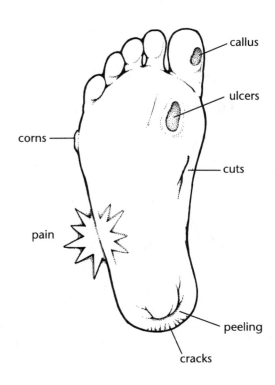

Keep your feet clean. Wash and dry them well. Don't forget to dry between your toes.

Keep your toenails trimmed. Trim your toenails to follow the curve of your toe. If you can't trim them yourself, have a member of your health care team do it.

Have your feet checked regularly. Take your shoes and socks off at every regular office visit to remind your doctor to check your feet. Have your doctor check your feet for blood vessel, muscle, and nerve damage at least once a year.

Keep blood glucose levels in your range. If blood glucose levels are high, you are more likely to get foot problems.

Keep your doctor informed. Call your doctor if you have a foot problem, no matter how minor.

Gestational Diabetes

Gestational diabetes is high blood glucose levels that occur only in pregnant women who do not already have diabetes. It appears around 24–28 weeks of pregnancy. At that time, the body is making large amounts of hormones to help the baby grow. It is thought that these hormones block insulin. When something in the body does not allow insulin to do its job, it is called insulin resistance.

In most pregnant women, the body makes enough insulin to overcome the insulin resistance. In other pregnant women, the insulin that is made cannot overcome the insulin resistance. These women have gestational diabetes. Most women with gestational diabetes have healthy babies. But close follow-up by a doctor is still important. You are at greater risk for gestational diabetes if one or more of the following statements are true:

- You are 25 years old or older.
- You are overweight.
- You have a family history of diabetes.
- You are Hispanic, Native American, African American, Asian, or a Pacific Islander.
- You have given birth to a baby weighing 9 pounds or more.

Gestational diabetes can be hard on you and your baby. If gestational diabetes is not treated, you and your baby are more likely to have the following problems.

MACROSOMIA

Macrosomia means large body. If your blood glucose is too high during pregnancy, the extra glucose in your blood goes into your baby. This causes your baby to make more insulin. The extra glucose and the extra insulin cause your baby to grow bigger and fatter than normal, making delivery harder. Babies who are larger than normal are more likely to have health problems and are more prone to diabetes later in life.

HYPOGLYCEMIA

Hypoglycemia is low blood glucose. If your blood glucose is too high right before or during labor, your baby may have low blood glucose at birth. The extra glucose in your blood goes into your baby. This causes your baby to make more insulin.

After delivery, your baby no longer gets extra glucose from you. The extra insulin your baby made causes your baby's blood glucose level to fall. Hypoglycemia in your baby can be treated in the hospital right after birth.

JAUNDICE

Before your baby is born, he or she makes lots of red blood cells. After delivery, your baby no longer needs as many red blood cells, and they are broken down. One breakdown product of red blood cells is bilirubin. Your baby's liver metabolizes the bilirubin. If your baby's liver is not mature enough, it may have trouble doing this. The extra red blood cells and bilirubin remain in your baby's body.

Bilirubin colors your baby's skin yellow. This is called jaundice. Jaundice can be taken care of in the hospital using special lights. It can be dangerous if it is not treated. Ask your doctor about it before you take your baby home from the hospital.

HIGH KETONES

Ketones are made when your body burns stored fat for energy. Large amounts of ketones can harm you or your baby. Testing your urine first thing in the morning can let you and your doctor know whether you are making too many ketones. Ketones are more likely to build up if you are not eating and drinking enough for both you and your baby. Be sure to eat all meals and snacks at your scheduled times.

PREECLAMPSIA

Preeclampsia (also called toxemia) is high blood pressure, swelling of your feet and lower legs, and leaking of protein into your urine during pregnancy. Other signs include headache, nausea, vomiting, abdominal pain, and blurred sight. If not treated, preeclampsia can cause seizures, coma, and death to you or your baby. Your doctor will watch for signs of preeclampsia.

URINARY TRACT INFECTION

When your blood glucose is high, you are more likely to get a urinary tract infection. Urinary tract infections are usually caused by bacteria. Bacteria grow much better and faster in high glucose.

Signs of a urinary tract infection include the need to urinate often, pain or burning when you urinate, cloudy or bloody urine, low back pain or abdominal pain, fever, and chills.

HOW TO CARE FOR GESTATIONAL DIABETES

If you are pregnant, get tested for gestational diabetes between the 24th and 28th weeks of pregnancy. If you have gestational diabetes, your doctor may ask you to meet with a diabetes educator who will help you learn to:

Follow a meal plan. A meal plan will help you avoid too high or too low blood glucose.

Follow an exercise program. Exercise can help lower your blood glucose level.

Self-monitor your blood glucose. This lets you know how your gestational diabetes care plan is working.

Check your urine for ketones. The earlier you detect ketones, the quicker you can stop them from getting worse. Ask your doctor when and how often you should check.

Take insulin. When you have gestational diabetes, your body may not be able to make and use all the insulin it needs for pregnancy. You may need to inject insulin. Diabetes pills are not used because they may harm the baby.

Gestational diabetes usually goes away after you give birth. But once you have had gestational diabetes, you are more likely to get type 2 diabetes in the future. Have your blood glucose checked (by the lab) at your 6-week follow-up visit with your doctor after your baby is born.

Health Care Team

A health care team is a group of health care professionals who help you manage your diabetes. The team includes you and may include a diabetes doctor (see Doctor), a diabetes educator nurse, a dietitian (see Dietitian), an exercise physiologist, a mental health professional, an eye doctor, a foot doctor, a dentist (see Dental Care), and a pharmacist. Your diabetes doctor may help you find the other members of the team.

Your team teaches you about diabetes and how to make diabetes care a part of your life. Your health care team depends on you to tell them how your diabetes care plan is working and when you need their help. That is why you are the most important member of the team.

DIABETES EDUCATOR NURSE

Nurses teach and advise you on the day-to-day management of your diabetes. Nurses can teach you what diabetes is and how to:

- Use diabetes pills
- Use insulin
- Give yourself insulin injections
- Use an insulin pump
- Check your blood glucose at home
- Keep track of your diabetes control
- Know the signs of low and high blood glucose

- Take care of low or high blood glucose
- Handle sick days
- Stay healthy during pregnancy

You may work with a diabetes nurse practitioner, a nurse clinician, or a nurse educator. Look for the initials RN after a nurse's name. RN stands for registered nurse. Some nurses also have a bachelor's degree (BSN) or a master's degree (MSN). Many nurses are certified diabetes educators (CDE). A certification for Advanced Practice nurses, dietitians, and pharmacists is indicated by BC-ADM (Board Certified, Advanced Diabetes Management).

CERTIFIED DIABETES EDUCATOR

The letters CDE after a person's name stand for certified diabetes educator. When you see these letters, you know the person is specially trained to teach or care for people with diabetes. These letters may come after the names of any of the people on your health care team.

A diabetes educator becomes certified by passing a test offered by the National Certification Board for Diabetes Educators—an independent organization established by the American Association of Diabetes Educators.

Once certified, CDEs must stay up-to-date on diabetes care and treatment in order to pass a recertification test every 5 years. To find a diabetes educator in your area, call the American Association of Diabetes Educators at 1-800-832-6874 or go to *www.aadenet.org*.

MENTAL HEALTH PROFESSIONAL

Mental health professionals include social workers, psychologists, and psychiatrists. These people can help you recognize and manage the emotional side of living with diabetes.

Look for a licensed clinical social worker (LCSW) with a master's degree in social work (MSW) and training in individual, group, and family therapy. Social workers can help you and your family cope with any stress or anxieties related to diabetes. They can help you locate community or government resources to help with medical or financial needs.

A clinical psychologist has a master's or doctoral degree in psychology and training in individual, group, and family psychotherapy. Clinical psychologists counsel patients with emotional problems.

A psychiatrist is a medical doctor who can provide counseling and prescribe drugs to treat physical causes for emotional problems.

EXERCISE PHYSIOLOGIST

An exercise physiologist is trained in the science of exercise and body conditioning. An exercise physiologist helps you plan a safe, effective exercise program.

Look for someone with a master's or doctoral degree in exercise physiology. Or find a licensed health care provider who has graduate training in exercise physiology. Certification from the American College of Sports Medicine is a good sign.

Always get your doctor's approval on any exercise program.

EYE DOCTOR

Your eye doctor is either an ophthalmologist or an optometrist. Ophthalmologists are medical doctors who detect and treat eye diseases. They may prescribe eye medicines and perform eye surgery. Optometrists are not medical doctors. They are trained to examine the eye for vision problems and other minor problems. When you go to an eye doctor, find out whether the eye doctor:

- Knows how to spot eye diseases
- Treats many patients with diabetes
- Performs eye surgery
- Will send regular reports to your diabetes doctor

FOOT DOCTOR

A foot doctor is called a podiatrist. A podiatrist is trained to treat foot and lower leg problems. Podiatrists have a doctor of podiatric medicine (DPM) degree from a college of podiatry. They have also done a residency (hospital training) in podiatry. When you go to a foot doctor, find out whether the foot doctor:

- Knows the foot problems diabetes can cause
- Treats many patients with diabetes
- Will work with your diabetes doctor

PHARMACIST

A pharmacist is trained in the chemistry of drugs and how drugs affect the body. A pharmacist has at least a bachelor of science in pharmacy degree (BScPharm) or a doctor of pharmacy degree (PharmD).

Your pharmacist can help you in several ways. Most pharmacists offer free counseling. They can tell you:

- How often to take your prescription drugs
- Whether to take your drugs with meals or on an empty stomach
- What side effects to watch for
- Whether to stay out of the sun
- What foods to avoid
- What other drugs might react with your new drug
- When to take a missed dose
- How to store your drugs
- What nonprescription drugs work best with your other drugs

OTHER TEAM MEMBERS

As your health changes, you may need other members on your team. If you plan to have a baby, you will need an obstetrician. If you have blood flow problems in your legs or feet, you may need a vascular surgeon. Your diabetes doctor can help you find the specialist you need.

Healthy Eating

A healthy eating plan is low in saturated fat and cholesterol, moderate in protein, high in starches and fiber, and moderate in sodium and sugars. This kind of eating can help protect you from heart disease, blood vessel damage, heart attack and stroke, colon and intestinal diseases, and some cancers.

LOW IN SATURATED FAT AND CHOLESTEROL

The two main kinds of fat in food are saturated fat and unsaturated fat. Saturated fat is highest in animal foods. Foods with a lot of saturated fat include meat, whole-milk dairy products, lard, shortening, and coconut and palm oils.

Saturated fats raise your cholesterol level more than anything else you eat. Cholesterol is found only in animal foods. Foods high in cholesterol include eggs, whole milk, regular cheeses, and meats.

Most plant foods are either low in fat or high in unsaturated fat. Unsaturated fats actually lower your cholesterol level. Unsaturated fats can be polyunsaturated or monounsaturated.

Vegetable oils, such as corn, cottonseed, safflower, soybean, and sunflower, are high in polyunsaturated fats. Oils that have mostly monounsaturated fats include olive, avocado, almond, canola, and peanut.

How to cut saturated fat and cholesterol

Dairy
- Use fat-free or reduced-fat milk in place of whole milk, half and half, or cream.
- Use plain low-fat or nonfat yogurt in place of cream, sour cream, or mayonnaise.
- Use pureed low-fat or nonfat cottage cheese with a little lemon juice in place of sour cream.
- Use low-fat or nonfat cream cheese or pureed low-fat or nonfat cottage cheese in place of regular cream cheese.
- Use low-fat or nonfat cheeses in place of regular cheeses.
- Use frozen low-fat or nonfat yogurt, ice cream, or sherbet in place of premium ice cream.

Eggs
- Limit whole eggs to three or four a week. You can use egg substitutes.
- In recipes, replace some of the whole eggs with egg whites. Two egg whites equal one whole egg.

Fats and oils
- Replace butter, regular margarine, lard, or shortening with soft tub, liquid, light, or diet margarine. You'll get less saturated fat.
- Replace butter or margarine with unsaturated oils. Try to cook food in a tablespoon or less of an unsaturated oil.
- Replace cooking oils with nonstick vegetable sprays, wine, or low-fat or nonfat broth.
- Replace regular oil-based salad dressings with low-fat or nonfat salad dressings. On salads, try lemon juice, or just salt and pepper, instead of dressing.

Meats
- Try to eat less meat. Keep your portion size to 3 oz—about the size of a deck of cards.

- Choose lean cuts of meat rather than fatty cuts. Some lean cuts include top round steak, eye round roast, pork tenderloin, lamb shank, and veal leg.
- Use low-fat cooking methods, such as grilling or broiling, instead of frying.

Poultry
- Choose chicken and turkey breast. They have the least amount of fat.
- Don't eat the skin.

Fish
- Try to eat more fish. Most fish are naturally low in fat and calories. Fish oils have omega-3 fatty acids, which may protect you from heart disease.
- Steam, poach, or grill your fish.

MODERATE IN PROTEIN

Protein is found in both animal and plant foods. For healthy eating, it's best to get your protein from foods that are low in fat, calories, and cholesterol.

Meats, eggs, milk, and cheese are high in protein. But they are also high in saturated fat and cholesterol. If you eat them, stick with lean cuts and low-fat versions.

Better choices for protein are chicken without skin, fish, and shellfish. Most fish and shellfish are lower in saturated fat and cholesterol than meat.

You can also get protein from legumes (beans, peas, and lentils), grains, and vegetables. These are good choices for protein because they are low in fat and calories and have no cholesterol.

Nuts and seeds have a good amount of protein in them, and most of the fat they contain is unsaturated.

HIGH IN STARCHES AND FIBER

Starches are one of the two major types of carbohydrate. (The other major type is sugar; see below.) Carbohydrate is the main nutrient in food that causes your blood glucose to rise. Starches include breads, cereals, pasta, rice, potatoes, corn, whole grains, dry beans, and peas. Most starches have very little fat or cholesterol.

Fiber, the part of plants that your body can't digest, is part of the total carbohydrate in a food. Fiber is found in fruits, vegetables, legumes (beans, peas, and lentils), and grains. All are low in fat and calories and have no cholesterol.

MODERATE IN SODIUM

Many foods contain salt as sodium. Foods high in sodium include canned foods, cured and smoked meats (bacon, sausage, salami, hot dogs, and bologna), pickles, cheeses, salad dressings, mustard, ketchup, soy sauce, breakfast cereals, frozen dinners, fast foods, and salty snacks (chips and pretzels).

How to cut sodium

- Choose low-sodium, reduced-sodium, or unsalted versions of foods.
- Rinse salted canned foods (such as vegetables, beans, fish, shellfish, and meats) with cold water for 1 minute to remove some of the sodium.
- Substitute chicken or turkey for prosciutto, ham, or other salty cured meats.
- Flavor your foods with lemon juice, flavored vinegars, peppers, garlic, onions, salt-free seasoning blends, and other herbs and spices in place of salt.

MODERATE IN SUGARS

Sugars are one of the two major types of carbohydrate. (The other major type is starch; see above.) Carbohydrate is the main nutrient in food that causes your blood glucose to rise.

Research has shown that sugars do not raise your blood glucose level any more than starches or other carbohydrates. Because of these findings, a moderate amount of sugars can be part of your healthy eating plan.

Sugars include honey, molasses, syrups (such as corn syrup and maple syrup), processed sugars (such as table sugar, brown sugar, and powdered sugar), and natural sugars (such as lactose in milk and fructose in fruits).

Foods with natural sugars are usually good sources of nutrients, such as vitamins, minerals, fiber, and protein. Many other nutritious foods, such as breakfast cereals, breads, and low-fat salad dressings, contain some added sugars. Some other foods with added sugar, such as chocolate, baked goods, and ice cream treats, provide lots of calories and fat with few nutrients.

Fructose may cause a smaller rise in your blood glucose level than other sugars. But large amounts of fructose may increase your cholesterol level. Because of this, there is no reason to use fructose in place of other sugars.

There is also no advantage to using fruit juice or fruit juice concentrates in place of other sugars. They provide just as many calories, and they raise blood glucose about as high as other sugars do.

Heart Attack

A heart attack occurs when blood flow to the muscle of the heart is stopped. Without blood, the heart can't get the oxygen it needs. Part of the heart muscle gets damaged or dies.

Blood flow can be cut off by a buildup of fat and cholesterol in the blood vessels (atherosclerosis) that lead to the heart. Or blood flow can be cut off by a clot stuck in one of the blood vessels.

People with diabetes are more likely to have a heart attack than people without diabetes. You can't change the fact that you have diabetes. But there are things you can do to keep your heart healthy.

HOW TO REDUCE YOUR RISK OF HEART ATTACK

- Control your diabetes. Keeping your blood glucose levels in your range (see Blood Glucose) and meeting your A1C goals (see A1C Test) may prevent or delay blood vessel damage.

- Toss the cigarettes. Smoking narrows blood vessels and promotes the buildup of fat and cholesterol on blood vessel walls. Smoking may even make your blood clot faster.

- If you have high blood pressure, work with your health care team to control it. High blood pressure makes your heart work harder. This weakens your heart. You can bring your blood pressure down by healthy eating, exercising, losing weight, and taking blood pressure drugs.

- Get a good low-fat, low-cholesterol cookbook and learn healthy, tasty ways to cook. High cholesterol can damage your blood vessels.

- Exercise for as little as 15 minutes a day three times a week, with a goal of working up to 30 minutes three times a week. Try walking, biking, or swimming. These and other aerobic exercises (see Exercise, Aerobic) can lower blood pressure, lower LDL cholesterol and triglycerides, and raise HDL cholesterol. Aerobic exercises can improve overall heart health, promote weight loss, and reduce stress.

- If you are overweight, lose a few pounds! Losing even a little weight with healthy eating and exercise lowers blood pressure and improves cholesterol levels.

- Know your lipid levels—HDL, LDL, and triglycerides.

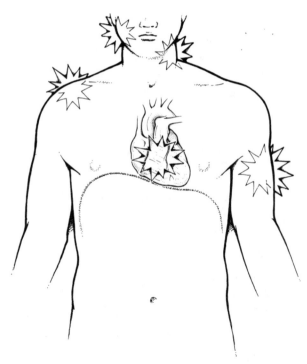

A heart attack may cause pain in the chest, neck, shoulders, arms, or jaw.

- Remain calm in the face of stress (see Relieve Stress). Excess stress can raise blood pressure and blood glucose levels.
- If you have gone through menopause, ask your doctor about the female hormone estrogen. Estrogen can have heart-healthy benefits. However, it is not without risks. Talk to your doctor about whether the benefits outweigh the risks for you.
- Be alert to the warning signs of a heart attack. Know what to do if the warning signs occur.

Warning signs of a heart attack

- Prolonged pain, tightness, pressure, or squeezing in the chest
- Pain that spreads to the neck, shoulders, arms, or jaw
- Shortness of breath or hiccups
- Dizziness or fainting
- Sweating
- Nausea

Special note: People with diabetes may have little or no pain.

IF YOU THINK YOU ARE HAVING A HEART ATTACK

1. Call 911 for an ambulance.
2. Tell those around you that you think you are having a heart attack. Otherwise, if you pass out, they may waste time trying to figure out what's wrong.

HHS

HS is an abbreviation for hyperosmolar hypergly-cemic nonketotic syndrome. It is a life-threatening state of high blood glucose and severe dehydration. Anyone with type 2 diabetes can develop HHS. But HHS doesn't just happen. It is usually brought on by something else, such as an illness or a heart attack.

In HHS, blood glucose levels rise, and your body tries to get rid of the excess glucose by passing it into your urine. Water is pulled from all over your body to dilute the glucose in your urine. As a result, you make lots of urine, and you have to urinate more often. You also get very thirsty. If you don't drink enough fluids at this point, you can get dehydrated.

If HHS continues, the severe dehydration will lead to seizures, coma, and eventually death. HHS usually takes days or even weeks to develop. Be alert to the warning signs of HHS.

WARNING SIGNS OF HHS

- Blood glucose level over 600 mg/dl
- Dry, parched mouth
- Extreme thirst (although this may gradually disappear)
- Warm, dry skin that does not sweat
- High fever (105°F, for example)
- Sleepiness or confusion

- Loss of vision
- Hallucinations
- Weakness on one side of the body

If you have any of these signs, call your doctor.

HOW TO AVOID HHS

The best way to avoid HHS is to check your blood glucose regularly. If you check your blood glucose once or twice a day, you will be alerted to high blood glucose before it worsens. When you are sick, check your blood glucose more often and drink a glassful of fluid (alcohol-free and caffeine-free) every hour.

High Blood Pressure

Blood pressure is the force of your blood as it travels through your blood vessels. The higher your blood pressure, the more force on your blood vessels. Added force on your blood vessels can weaken and damage them.

Blood vessels nourish your organs and nerves. When blood vessels are weakened and damaged by high blood pressure, they don't nourish your organs and nerves as well as they should. Your organs and nerves become damaged.

People with diabetes are more likely to have high blood pressure than people without diabetes. High blood pressure increases your chances of having a heart attack or stroke (see Heart Attack; and Stroke) and may worsen nephropathy (kidney disease) and retinopathy (an eye disease).

SIGNS OF HIGH BLOOD PRESSURE

High blood pressure usually has no signs. The only way to know whether you have it is to get it checked. Your blood pressure is probably checked each time you visit your doctor.

Checking your blood pressure

Blood pressure can be checked with a device called a sphygmomanometer. A soft cuff is wrapped around your upper arm. The cuff is inflated until it tightens enough to stop the flow of blood. As the cuff is deflated, the force of the blood is heard through a stethoscope.

Blood pressure is reported as two numbers. The first number is the systolic pressure. Systolic pressure is the force of your blood when your heart contracts. The second number is the diastolic pressure. Diastolic pressure is the force of your blood when your heart relaxes.

A reading of "120 over 80" means a systolic pressure of 120 and a diastolic pressure of 80. It is written as 120/80 mmHg (millimeters [mm] of mercury [Hg]).

Hypertension is another name for high blood pressure. If you find out that your blood pressure is high, you and your health care team can take steps to control it. Your doctor will first try to find out the cause of your high blood pressure.

	Blood Pressure Reading (in mmHg)
Normal blood pressure	Less than 120/80
Prehypertension	121/81 to 139/89
Stage 1 hypertension	140/90 to 159/99
Stage 2 hypertension	More than 160/100

Adapted from The U.S. Department of Health and Human Services, *The Seventh Report of the Joint National Committee on Prevention, Detection, Evaluation, and Treatment of High Blood Pressure* (Washington, D.C., 2003).

CAUSES OF HIGH BLOOD PRESSURE

Sometimes, there is a specific cause, such as a kidney problem, hormone disorder, pregnancy, or the use of birth control pills. When high blood pressure is linked to a specific cause, it is called secondary hypertension. If you have secondary hypertension, your doctor will treat the cause first.

Most of the time, there is no obvious cause for high blood pressure. When there is no obvious cause, it is called essential hypertension. If you have essential hypertension, there are things you can do to bring your blood pressure down without having to take drugs.

HOW TO LOWER YOUR BLOOD PRESSURE

Lose excess weight. Losing even a little extra weight may be enough to return your blood pressure to normal. The only way to lose weight and to keep it off is to follow a weight-loss plan. Your health care team can help you make a plan that you can live with.

Stop smoking. Smoking causes high blood pressure by damaging blood vessels. Stopping smoking can do more to lower your risk of hypertension-related death than taking blood pressure drugs.

Drink less alcohol. Drinking more than 2 oz of alcohol a day may cause high blood pressure. Your doctor may advise you to drink no more than 1 oz of alcohol a day. There is about 1 oz of alcohol in one mixed drink, one glass of wine, or a can of beer.

Eat less salt. Avoiding your salt shaker and foods with added salt may be enough to lower your blood pressure. If your doctor wants you to try a low-sodium diet, plan one with a registered dietitian.

Reduce stress. Stress may aggravate high blood pressure by causing your blood vessels to constrict and your heart to work harder. For tips on reducing stress, see Relieve Stress.

If you are not able to bring your blood pressure down by these changes, your doctor will likely put you on drugs to lower your blood pressure.

Blood pressure drugs used most often in people with diabetes are ACE (angiotensin-converting enzyme) inhibitors, ARBs (angiotensin-receptor blockers), calcium antagonists, and thiazide diuretics in small doses.

These blood pressure drugs do not raise blood glucose levels, but they all have side effects. Ask your doctor or pharmacist about them.

Insulin

nsulin is a hormone that helps glucose get inside your body's cells. Your cells use glucose for energy. Insulin is made in the pancreas. Your pancreas lies behind your stomach.

If you have type 1 diabetes, your pancreas no longer makes insulin, or it makes only a tiny amount. That's why you need to take insulin.

If you have type 2 diabetes, your pancreas still makes insulin. But it doesn't make enough, or your body has a hard time using the insulin, or both. You may need to take diabetes pills or you may need to take insulin.

INSULIN ACTION

Insulin's action has three parts: onset, peak, and duration. Onset is how long insulin takes to start working. Peak is when insulin is working its hardest. Duration is how long insulin keeps working.

The times for onset, peak, and duration are given as ranges in the following table. The main reason for these ranges is that insulin may work slower or faster in you than in someone else.

INSULIN ACTION

Type	Onset (hours)	Peak (hours)	Effective Duration (hours)	Maximum Duration (hours)
Aspart	0.25	0.5–1.5	2–4	4–6
Lispro	0.25	0.5–1.5	2–4	4–6
Regular	0.5–1	2–3	3–6	6–10
NPH	2–4	4–10	10–16	14–18
Lente	3–4	4–12	12–18	16–20
Ultralente	6–10	—	18–20	20–24
Glargine	3–5	No peak	24	24

INSULIN STRENGTH

Insulins come dissolved in liquids. Most people use U-100 insulin. This means that there are 100 units of insulin per milliliter of fluid. If you inject insulin, it is important to use a syringe that matches the strength of your insulin. For instance, if you use U-100 insulin, use a U-100 syringe.

INSULIN STORAGE

Insulin makers advise storing your insulin in the refrigerator before being opened. Do not put your insulin in the freezer or allow it to warm in the sun. Extreme temperatures can destroy insulin. Most doctors believe the bottle of insulin you are using can be left at room temperature for up to a month.

INSULIN SAFETY

Check the expiration date before opening your insulin. If the date has passed, don't use the insulin. If the date is yet to come, look closely at the insulin in the bottle. If you are looking at insulin aspart, insulin lispro, insulin glargine, or regular insulin, it should be clear, with no particles or color. If you are looking at NPH, lente, or ultralente insulin, it should be cloudy. But it should not have particles or crystals.

If the insulin does not look as it should, return the unopened bottle of insulin to the place you bought it for an exchange or refund.

INSULIN THERAPY

Your doctor will help you plan what kinds of insulin to take, how much, and when. It is important to follow this plan closely. Your plan may be a standard or an intensive one.

Standard insulin therapy means you inject insulin one or two times a day at the same dose and same times each day. Often, you give yourself one injection in the morning and one in the evening.

Standard therapy may work well for you, or it may leave your blood glucose levels too high. But you usually won't have severe high or low blood glucose levels.

Intensive insulin therapy means you inject insulin three or more times a day or use an insulin pump. You change your insulin dose to fit the results of your blood glucose checks, how much you are planning to eat, or what exercises or activities you are going to do.

Intensive therapy aims to keep your blood glucose levels very close to normal. Because you are keeping your blood glucose levels lower, your chances of having severe low blood glucose are greater. You may also gain some weight.

Talk with your health care team about which insulin therapy is best for you. The best therapy is the one that helps you meet your blood glucose and A1C test goals.

Insulin Injections

nsulin cannot be taken in a pill. It would be broken down like food before it could work. Insulin needs to be injected under the skin, in the fat, to work well. Injecting into fat is much less painful than injecting into muscle. Besides, if you inject into muscle, the insulin will not work as well. Usually it will work too fast.

WHERE TO INJECT INSULIN

When choosing a place to inject insulin, consider the area and the site. Areas are the places on your body where it is good to inject insulin. Four good areas are your:

1. Abdomen (anywhere except within 2 inches of your navel)
2. Upper arms (outside part)
3. Buttocks (anywhere)
4. Thighs (front and outside parts, not inner thigh, not right above your knee)

These areas absorb insulin at different speeds. Your abdomen absorbs insulin the fastest, followed by the arms, buttocks, and thighs. You may prefer to inject insulin in the same area so that you know how it will act. Or you may want to choose your area according to how fast or slow you want the insulin to start working.

One plan is to inject your breakfast and lunch insulin doses into your arms and abdomen (the areas that absorb faster)

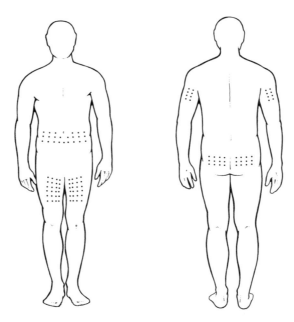

Sites for insulin shots

and to inject your supper and bedtime doses into your buttocks and thighs (the areas that absorb slower). Your doctor may suggest another plan for you. Whatever plan you try, keep track of how your body responds by checking your blood glucose and recording the results.

Now pretend that each area is covered with circles that are 1 inch apart. Each circle is one site. The number of sites you have depends on how big your body is. The bigger your body, the more sites you have in each area.

Within each area, it is best to change sites with each injection. This is called site rotation. To rotate sites, you use a different circle for each injection until all the circles have been used up. Then you start all over again. If you take all your injections in the same place, you can damage the tissue under your skin.

HOW TO INJECT INSULIN

1. Wash your hands with soap and water. Dry them.
2. Clean the site.

3. Wipe the top of the insulin vial with 70% isopropyl alcohol.

4. Gently roll the vial in your hands to mix the insulin. (You do not need to do this to lispro or regular insulin.)

5. Draw air into the syringe. Stop at the mark for the insulin dose you want. Inject the air into the vial. This prevents a vacuum.

6. Turn the bottle upside down. Draw insulin into the syringe. Stop at the mark for the number of units you want. When mixing types of insulin, draw the shorter-acting insulin first.

7. Check for air bubbles. If there are air bubbles, flick your forefinger against the upright syringe a couple of times to get them out.

8. Gently grasp a fold of skin between your thumb and forefinger.

9. Push the needle through the skin at a 90-degree angle. If you are thin, you may need to push the needle in at a 45-degree angle to avoid muscle.

10. After the needle is in, push the plunger to inject the insulin.

11. Pull the needle out.

HOW TO MAKE THE INJECTION MORE COMFORTABLE

Syringes for injecting insulin have tiny needles with a slick coating so that they go in easily. Most people find that insulin injections don't hurt too much, if done correctly.

• Inject insulin at room temperature. Using cold insulin right from the refrigerator may make it hurt more.

• Make sure there are no air bubbles in the syringe before you inject the insulin.

• Relax your muscles in the area.

• Puncture the skin quickly.

• Keep the needle going in the same direction when you put it in and take it out.

• Use sharp, not dull, needles.

HOW TO REUSE SYRINGES

Makers of disposable syringes recommend that they be used only once. The makers cannot guarantee that the syringe will stay sterile. If you want to use your syringes more than once, check with your doctor first.

- Recap the needle after each use to keep it clean.
- Keep the needle from touching anything but clean skin and your insulin vial stopper.
- Store the used syringe at room temperature.
- Throw away the syringe when the needle is dull, has been bent, or has come into contact with any surface other than your skin or insulin vial stopper.
- Don't try to clean the needle with alcohol. Alcohol may remove the slick coating that makes injections less painful.
- Watch out for infection at the site.

HOW TO DISPOSE OF SYRINGES

The best way to dispose of syringes and needles is to place them in a puncture-proof container of heavy-duty plastic or metal with a screw cap or other lid that can be sealed shut before it is placed in the garbage.

Another way to dispose of needles is with a needle-clipping device that clips, catches, and keeps the needles in a closed compartment.

Some states require you to destroy used insulin syringes and needles. But be careful if you recap, bend, or break a needle—you or someone else could get pricked with it.

There may be special rules for getting rid of syringes and needles where you live. Ask your local garbage company or city or county waste authority what method meets their rules.

Insulin Pumps

An insulin pump is a battery-powered, computerized device about the size of a pager. Inside the pump is a vial of insulin with a gear-driven plunger. A thin tube, 21 to 43 inches long, is attached to the pump. At the other end of the tube is a needle or catheter. You insert the needle or catheter under your skin, usually in your abdomen or thigh. Insulin is delivered through the tube and needle or catheter into your body.

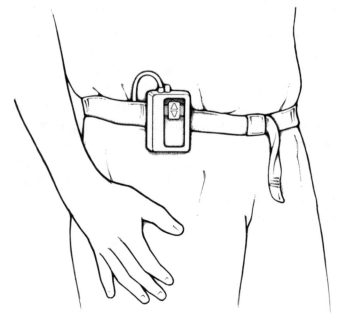

Insulin Pump

You program the pump. You tell it how much insulin you want and when you want it. You tell the pump to give you tiny amounts of insulin continuously throughout the day and night (basal), just the way a normal pancreas would. Then you tell the pump to give you extra insulin just before you eat (bolus).

You wear an insulin pump pretty much all the time, either inside or outside your clothes. A pump may be waterproof or come with a waterproof case for showers and swimming.

You can, of course, take the pump off. If you'll have the pump off for more than 1 hour, you may need an injection of insulin. Check your blood glucose to be sure. Yes, you still need to check your blood glucose. At least four times a day is recommended.

WHAT THE PUMP CAN DO FOR YOU

Get your blood glucose levels closer to normal. This is called tight control. If your insulin injections have not controlled your blood glucose levels, an insulin pump might work better for you.

Smooth out blood glucose swings. If you have frequent blood glucose swings, the insulin pump can help smooth them out.

Take care of nighttime lows and morning highs. Your body needs less insulin at night than at dawn. If you try to lower the dose of your injected evening insulin to avoid low blood glucose at night, you won't have enough insulin in the morning. Then you'll have high blood glucose when you wake up.

With an insulin pump, you can program it to give you less insulin at night and more insulin before dawn. That way you avoid nighttime low blood glucose and morning high blood glucose.

BE AWARE

Ketoacidosis. When your body has too little or no insulin, you risk getting ketoacidosis. Ketoacidosis is a dangerous buildup of ketones in your blood.

If the tube to your insulin pump gets blocked or twisted or the needle comes out, you won't be getting insulin and you may not know it. (Pumps do have alarms that signal when the tube is blocked, the insulin is low, or the battery is low. But they don't signal when the needle has come out.)

Ketones can start to build up in 1 hour. Ketoacidosis can develop in as little as 6 hours. Your best protection is to check your blood glucose levels often. If your blood glucose level is above 250 mg/dl, check your urine for ketones.

Infection. The place where the needle or catheter enters your body may become infected. To lessen your chances of infection, clean the area before you insert the needle or catheter, change sites within the area every 48 hours (see Insulin Injections), and use an antibiotic ointment and protective cover.

Skin allergy. You may have an allergic reaction around the needle or catheter site. Try nonallergenic tape or Teflon catheters.

Insurance

Diabetes can be costly, so finding the best possible health insurance coverage is important. Health insurance plans and policies vary greatly on what costs they will cover. Before you sign up for a health insurance plan, find the answers to these questions:

- How much is the monthly premium and what are the co-payments for each service or item covered by the policy?
- Does the plan have a preexisting exclusion that will make you pay (usually for 6 or 12 months) before receiving coverage for diabetes needs?
- Are visits to your diabetes doctor covered? How many visits are allowed? How much will you have to pay at each visit?
- What supplies are covered? Are there co-payments, cost limits, or restrictions on the amount of supplies you can purchase? Are you required to buy your supplies through a pharmacy or a durable medical equipment provider?
- Does the plan cover diabetes education or the services of a dietitian?
- What mental health benefits are covered?
- Does the plan cover the services of specialists, such as an endocrinologist, eye doctor, podiatrist, or dentist?
- What medications are paid for? Is there a prescription plan? How often can prescriptions be refilled? Is a co-payment required for each prescription? Are you

required to fill your diabetes prescriptions through mail order or can your local pharmacy fill your prescriptions?

- Is home health care and nursing home coverage included? Are there any limitations?

GROUP COVERAGE

If you're employed, you may have the option of joining a group policy offered by your employer. If an employer grants insurance to one employee, it must offer the same policy to all employees. The health plan may require you to reveal your health history before covering some or all of your diabetes needs if this is your first time purchasing insurance through a group, or if you were uninsured for a long time before enrolling. Fees for group insurance vary. Many policies will also cover your spouse and children for an additional fee. Health care is nontaxable, so if you pay a fee, you may deduct it from your paycheck before taxes are taken out. If your employer does not offer health in- surance, you may still be able to obtain group insurance through membership in a professional, trade, or religious association.

INDIVIDUAL COVERAGE

If you are not eligible for group insurance, you may try to find an individual health insurance policy. Unfortunately, this can be difficult for a person with diabetes and the cost can be very expensive, often with fewer benefits than offered in a group plan. Also, most states allow health insurers to charge more for individual health insurance policies that cover people with diabetes (New York, New Jersey, Ver- mont, Massachusetts, Pennsylvania, Hawaii, and Michigan have laws to protect against this).

Check to see if your state has a high-risk health insurance pool available to people with diseases like diabetes. Though the require- ments to qualify for high-risk pools are sometimes difficult and the policies may be expensive, many states do make high-risk pools avail- able to people with chronic conditions.

TYPES OF HEALTH INSURANCE

Fee-for-service plans

In a fee-for-service plan, you and/or your employer pay a yearly or monthly fee called a premium. The insurance company then pays for all or part of your medical care. Usually, the insurer will start paying after you pay a small amount of the cost (the deductible). You may also have to pay a small amount (co-pay) for visits or healthcare. An advantage of a fee-for-service plan is that you pick the health care providers you want to go to.

Managed care plans

Under a managed care plan, you must obtain your health care from a specified group of health care providers unless you want to pay more for services provided by someone outside of the group. Types of managed care plans include health maintenance organizations (HMOs), preferred provider organizations (PPOs), and exclusive provider organizations (EPOs).

Like a fee-for-service plan, you and/or your employer pay a yearly or monthly premium. The insurance company then pays for all or part of your medical care. If you go to a doctor who is not a member of your managed care group, you'll have to pay more for service—maybe the entire bill. You may also have to pay a co-pay for visits or healthcare to providers within your group.

CONSOLIDATED OMNIBUS BUDGET RECONCILIATION ACT (COBRA)

Under COBRA, your employer must allow you to keep an equal health insurance policy for up to 18 months after you leave your job. You will have to pay for the coverage and may be charged up to 2 percent extra, but this is usually less expensive than paying for a new short-term policy on your own. If you are disabled, you can be covered by COBRA for 29 months. Dependents can continue their coverage for up to 36 months. Once you have been laid off or leave a company, you have 60 days to accept COBRA benefits. During that 60 days, your employer must pay insurance bills for you or your dependents. Employers with fewer than 20 employees, the federal government, employers that go out of business, and churches are exempt from COBRA, though they may still offer COBRA to employees.

If you are not eligible for COBRA, or if your COBRA coverage runs out, you still have options. Many states require employers to offer you a conversion policy regardless of your health or physical condition, usually at a higher cost and with less benefits (15 states and the District of Columbia do not require this). However, it may be your only choice and is better than going without insurance. Once your COBRA insurance runs out or you leave your job, you have 31 days to accept or reject a conversion plan. For more on COBRA, call the COBRA hotline at 202-219-8776.

HEALTH INSURANCE PORTABILITY AND ACCOUNTABILITY ACT OF 1996

According to this law, insurers and employers may not make insurance rules that discriminate against workers because of their health. All workers eligible for a certain health insurance plan must be offered enrollment at the same price. Insurers who sell individual policies must offer an individual policy without preexisting condition exclusions to anyone who has had continuous coverage in a group plan for the previous 18 months, is not currently eligible for coverage under a group plan, and has used up COBRA coverage.

The law also helps you keep coverage when you change jobs. If you have had diabetes for more than 6 months and have had continuous coverage in an insurance plan and then leave your job, you cannot be denied coverage by your new employer because of a preexisting condition. If, however, you have been recently diagnosed (within 6 months) and you change jobs, your new employer may refuse or limit your health insurance coverage for a year. This is a one-time waiting period, and it can be reduced by the number of months you had coverage at your previous job since your diagnosis.

MEDICARE

Medicare is a federal health insurance program for people over the age of 65 and for some people with disabilities who can't work. Even with Medicare, you may still have to pay for a large part of your medical bills. You can sign up for Medicare 3 months before the month of your 65th birthday.

There are 2 parts to Medicare—Part A and Part B. Part A helps pay for medical care provided in hospitals, skilled nursing facilities, hospices (for people who are dying), and nursing homes. It will not cover custodial care (help with daily activities, such as walking, getting dressed, etc.) if that is the only care you need.

Though most people covered by Medicare get Part A, Part B (available for a monthly fee) is critical, especially if you have diabetes. Part B helps pay for health providers' services, ambulance services, diagnostic tests, outpatient hospital services, outpatient physical therapy, speech pathology services, and medical equipment and supplies. Coverage has expanded to include diabetes education, nutrition services, and many diabetes supplies. Your doctor must certify in writing that you need all of these items to manage your diabetes. Make copies of this written statement and give a copy to your pharmacist each time you purchase supplies.

There are many diabetes-related services and supplies Medicare will and won't pay for. To learn more about Medicare, call 1-800-MEDICARE (633-4227) and ask for a copy of *Medicare Coverage of Diabetes Supplies and Services,* or visit *www.medicare.gov* to get the information online. For a detailed explanation of Medicare, get a free copy of *Your Medicare Handbook* from the Social Security Administration at 1-800-772-1213.

MEDIGAP AND MEDICARE HMOs

Medigap plans are sold by private insurance companies to cover some of the charges that Medicare won't. Medicare HMOs usually replace traditional Medicare policies and require you to go to a select group of health care providers. You cannot be denied Medigap if you apply within 6 months of first applying for Medicare Part B. You can't be denied a Medicare HMO as long as you select the policy during a period known as open enrollment that happens at least once a year. Be sure to read the policy carefully and shop around before purchasing.

The booklet *Guide to Health Insurance for People with Medicare*, is updated every year and is available through any insurance company or through Social Security. It contains the ever-changing federal standards for Medigap policies and general information about Medicare.

MEDICAID

If your income is very low, or you're disabled, a senior citizen, or a child, you might be able to get Medicaid. Medicaid is a federal and state assistance program. Each state decides what income level it thinks is very low and each state decides what medical services and supplies to cover. Call your state's Medicaid office to find out whether you qualify and what health costs are covered.

SOCIAL SECURITY DISABILITY INSURANCE

If you lose your job because you are disabled, you may be able to get this insurance. This insurance covers people younger than age 65 who have worked for pay recently and who are now disabled. Social Security has a list of disabilities. If you have a disability on that list and earn less than $800 a month, you are considered disabled. The disabilities that are listed include diabetes with certain kinds of neuropathy, acidosis, amputation, or retinopathy. For more information, call Social Security on weekdays at 1-800-772-1213.

Juvenile Diabetes Rights

Children with diabetes must be medically safe while at school and day care and also have the same access to educational opportunities as other children. The best way to ensure good diabetes care for your child is to communicate openly with school personnel and to make sure staff members understand their roles in meeting your child's medical needs. It is also important for you to understand your rights and what you can do to make sure your child receives fair treatment and appropriate care.

LAWS

The Rehabilitation Act of 1973 protects individuals with disabilities against discrimination in any program or activity receiving federal funds. This includes all public schools and day care centers, and private schools and centers that receive federal assistance. Schools can lose federal funding if they do not comply with this law. The Americans with Disabilities Act prohibits all schools and day care centers, except those run by religious organizations, from discriminating against children with disabilities. The Individuals with Disabilities Education Act protects a child with a disability who can show that the disability adversely affects his or her educational performance. Once shown, parents and school officials develop an Individualized Education Program (IEP). In addition to these federal laws, some state laws provide even more protection.

YOUR RIGHTS

As a parent or legal guardian of a child with diabetes, you have the right to have your child assessed, to hold a meeting with school personnel, to develop an education plan that specifically states what services will be provided to meet your child's needs, and to be notified of any proposed changes to your child's plan and to approve any changes.

DIABETES MEDICAL MANAGEMENT PLAN

It is important for you, your child's health care team, and school personnel to work together to ensure a medically safe environment for your child, while making sure he or she is able to fully participate in all school-sponsored activities. Your child's health care team should work with you to develop a Diabetes Medical Management Plan that enables school personnel to carry out the diabetes care regimen prescribed by your child's health care team.

EDUCATION PLAN TO MEET NEEDS

In addition to the Diabetes Medical Management Plan, services required to meet your child's needs should be documented in an education plan, such as an IEP. The plan should outline your child's academic and medical needs (in accordance with the Diabetes Medical Management Plan) and state the services that will be provided to these needs. Your written plan may include requirements such as:

- Assuring the on-site availability of trained personnel
- Allowing your child to self-administer and self-treat
- Ensuring full participation in all school activities including sports, extracurricular events, and field trips
- Immediate access to diabetes supplies and snacks
- Extra trips to the bathroom and water fountain
- Permitting extra absences for medical appointments and sick days

ADDRESSING DISCRIMINATION

If you believe your child has been discriminated against and is not receiving appropriate diabetes care from his or her school, the best course of action is first educate, then negotiate, litigate, and, if necessary, legislate.

Educate. Discrimination based on diabetes is often the result of ignorance. It is important to educate school personnel about diabetes and how it affects your child.

Negotiate. When education alone is not enough, try to negotiate a resolution to the problem.

Litigate. If your child's needs are not being met, you have the right to file an administrative complaint or a lawsuit in court.

Legislate. If you find the current laws and policies are not providing your child with the needed protection, your next step might be working to change the rules at a local, statewide, or national level.

If you want more information about your child's rights at school or day care, call 1-800-DIABETES for the ADA's packet on school discrimination or to discuss a specific school or day care problem with ADA's Legal Advocate.

Kidney Disease

Kidneys clean your blood. Your blood flows through filters in your kidneys. In healthy kidneys, the filters let wastes pass out to your urine while keeping good and useful things in your blood. But having diabetes can make your kidneys unhealthy. Unhealthy kidneys can get kidney disease. Kidney disease is also called nephropathy.

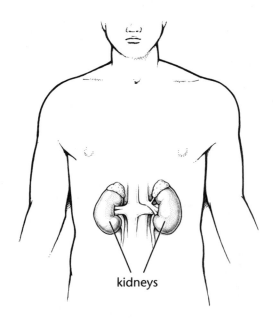

kidneys

Kidneys are located on either side of the small of your back.

THE PROGRESS OF KIDNEY DISEASE

In kidney disease, kidneys go from being overworked, to leaky, to not being able to filter, and finally, to failure.

Overworked filters. People with diabetes often have high levels of glucose in their blood. High levels of glucose make your kidneys filter blood more often than is really needed. This extra work can be hard on the filters. The filters can become overworked.

Leaky filters. Overworked filters may start to leak. One thing they can leak is a protein called albumin. The filters leak albumin into the urine. A small amount of albumin in the urine is the first outward sign of kidney damage. As more and more albumin leaks into the urine, the level of albumin in the blood falls.

Very leaky filters. One job of albumin is to hold water in the blood. If there is not enough albumin in the blood, water leaks out of the blood vessels. The water can end up in the ankles, the abdomen, and the chest.

Water in your ankles makes them swell. Water in your abdomen causes bloating. Water in your chest makes it hard to breathe. These may be the first physical signs that something is wrong with your kidneys. But they are late signs of kidney disease.

Filters that don't filter well. After a time, some of the overworked leaky filters just stop working. This makes more work for the filters that are still good. At first, the good filters work harder to make up for the ones that have stopped. Then they, too, stop working.

As more filters stop, fewer filters are left to do the work. Eventually, none of the filters are able to remove wastes. Wastes build up in the blood.

Filters that fail. Wastes in the blood rise to toxic levels when the kidneys' filters are no longer working. This is called kidney failure or end-stage renal disease.

SIGNS OF KIDNEY FAILURE

Foul taste in the mouth	Easy bruising
Poor appetite	Restless legs
Upset stomach	Loss of sleep at night
Throwing up	Lack of concentration

A person with kidney failure needs to have either a kidney transplant or dialysis. In a kidney transplant, the person gets a new kidney from someone else. In dialysis, a solution or a machine cleans the blood. There are steps you can take to slow down kidney disease before kidney failure.

HOW TO SLOW DOWN KIDNEY DISEASE

Keep your blood glucose levels close to normal. Keeping your blood glucose levels close to normal is known as tight control. Tight blood glucose control, more than anything else, can slow the progress of kidney disease.

Have your doctor check how your kidneys are working. There are urine tests and blood tests to detect the start and progress of kidney disease. Two blood tests (blood urea nitrogen and serum creatinine) and one urine test (creatinine clearance) tell how well your kidneys are getting rid of wastes. Another urine test for microalbumin shows whether your kidneys are leaking. You should have this test once a year.

Keep an eye on your blood pressure. When your kidneys' filters are not working well, extra salt and water stay in the body. This can raise blood pressure. High blood pressure makes the kidneys work harder, and they can get more damaged.

If you have high blood pressure, try to get it under 130/80. Some ways to bring blood pressure down are by losing weight, eating less salt, and avoiding alcohol.

Ask your doctor about drugs to lower blood pressure. Two classes of blood pressure drugs, called ACE (angiotensin-converting enzyme) inhibitors and ARBs (angiotensin-receptor blockers), may even slow the progress of kidney disease.

Limit protein. Some researchers have found that if you limit the amount of protein you eat, you may slow down kidney disease. But experts have not agreed on how much protein is best.

Most Americans get about 14 to 18 percent of their daily calories from protein. The American Diabetes Association recommends that people with signs of kidney disease get about 10 percent of their daily calories from protein.

Foods high in protein include meat, fish, poultry, eggs, milk, cheese, legumes, whole grains, and nuts and seeds. Work with a dietitian to make a low-protein meal plan, if needed.

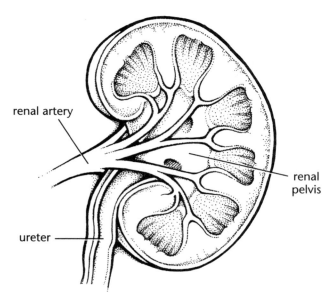

renal artery

renal pelvis

ureter

Detail of a kidney

Lipids

Lipids is another word for blood fats. Fats are part of every cell in your body. Fats include cholesterol and triglycerides. Both cholesterol and triglycerides are made by your body. You can also get cholesterol from the animal foods you eat.

Your body uses cholesterol to build cell walls and to make certain vitamins and hormones. Your body uses triglycerides as stored fat. Stored fat keeps you warm, protects your body's organs, and gives you energy reserves.

Cholesterol and triglycerides travel through your body in your blood. These two blood fats can only travel by being carried. They are carried by lipoproteins (lipo means fat), which is why they're referred to as lipids. Three kinds of lipids are:

1. Very-low-density lipoprotein (VLDL). VLDL carries triglycerides, cholesterol, and other fats. VLDL drops off triglycerides and other fats in fat tissue. VLDL then becomes LDL.

2. Low-density lipoprotein (LDL). LDL carries cholesterol to parts of the body that need it. Along the way, LDL cholesterol can stick to blood vessel walls. Cholesterol on blood vessel walls can lead to atherosclerosis or hardening of the arteries. The less LDL in your blood, the better.

3. High-density lipoprotein (HDL). HDL carries cholesterol away from the blood vessel walls to the liver. The liver breaks down the cholesterol and sends it out of the body. The more HDL in your blood, the better.

People with diabetes often have high lipid levels. High lipid levels put you at risk for heart disease, heart attack, and stroke. If you want to reduce your risk, first find out what your lipid levels are.

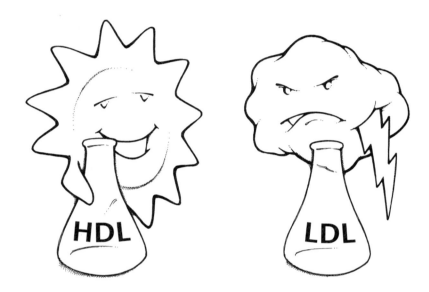

THE HEALTHIEST LIPID LEVELS

- Total cholesterol under 200 mg/dl
- LDL cholesterol under 100 mg/dl
- HDL cholesterol over 40 mg/dl for men and over 50 mg/dl for women
- Triglycerides under 150 mg/dl

If your lipid levels match these, great! If your lipid levels do not match these, try the following steps.

HOW TO IMPROVE LIPID LEVELS

- First, control your diabetes. Controlling your diabetes means keeping your blood glucose in a range set by your doctor. When your diabetes is out of control, it is harder to improve lipid levels.

- Lose weight if you need to. Extra weight makes it harder to control blood glucose and can raise total cholesterol. Besides, losing weight raises your good HDL cholesterol.

- Start cutting back on saturated fat (see Healthy Eating). Your liver uses the fat you eat to make VLDL. The more fat you eat, the more VLDL the liver makes. More VLDL means more bad LDL cholesterol.

- Replace saturated fats (butter, lard) with monounsaturated fats (canola and olive oil). Saturated fats raise your LDL and total cholesterol levels. Monounsaturated fats lower them.

- Eat fewer high-cholesterol foods. Foods high in cholesterol include organ meats, such as liver, and egg yolks. If you eat eggs every day, try cutting back to three or four a week. You can also try using just the egg whites or an egg substitute.

- Eat more high-fiber foods. Soluble fiber helps remove cholesterol from the body. Oats, beans, peas, fresh fruits, and brown rice are great fiber choices.

- Take a hike or go for a walk. Aerobic exercises, such as brisk walking, jogging, swimming, and skiing, raise your good HDL cholesterol. Find exercises you enjoy.

- If you smoke, cut down or quit. Smoking lowers your good HDL cholesterol.

- Take the medication prescribed by your doctor.

Have your lipid levels checked at least once a year or more often if your doctor recommends.

Meal Planning

Most people with diabetes have a meal plan. A meal plan tells you what to eat, how much to eat, and when to eat. A dietitian can help you make a meal plan that is right for you. It should be based on:

- What you like to eat and drink
- When you like to eat and drink
- How many calories you need
- Your level of activity
- What exercises you do
- When you exercise
- Your health
- What medications you take
- Your family or cultural customs

A typical meal plan includes breakfast, lunch, supper, and a bedtime snack. You may also have snacks at midmorning and midafternoon. Your meal plan can include special meal plans for sick days, pregnancy, and travel.

Diabetes meal plans are healthy. A healthy meal plan includes a variety of foods: grains, fruits, vegetables, legumes, dairy products, meats, and fats.

Being consistent is a big part of diabetes meal planning, especially if you take insulin. Try to eat the same number of calories, the same amounts of food, and the same kinds of foods at the same times each day, or vary your insulin accordingly.

Doing this helps you control your blood glucose levels. If you skip a meal or snack, you risk large swings in your blood glucose levels.

A meal plan can help you meet your other health goals as well. Your other health goals may include:

- Better blood fat levels
- Normal blood pressure
- A healthy weight

Three meal-planning tools for people with diabetes are exchange lists, carbohydrate counting, and the food pyramid.

EXCHANGE LISTS

Exchange lists are lists of foods grouped together because they are alike. One serving of any of the foods on a list has about the same amount of carbohydrate, protein, fat, and calories. Any food on a list may be "exchanged" or traded for any other food on the same list.

Your dietitian can help you work out a plan using the exchange lists. The meal plan will tell you the number of food exchanges you can eat at each meal and snack. You then choose foods that add up to those exchanges. When choosing foods, be aware that the serving size on a food label may not be the same as the serving size of an exchange.

With exchange lists, as long as you follow your plan, you are eating a balanced diet. In *Exchange Lists for Meal Planning*, published by the American Diabetes Association and The American Dietetic Association, there are 15 exchange lists.

CARBOHYDRATES
1. Starches
2. Fruit
3. Milk
4. Sweets, Desserts, and Other Carbohydrates
5. Nonstarchy Vegetables

MEAT AND MEAT SUBSTITUTES
6. Very-Lean
7. Lean
8. Medium-Fat
9. High-Fat

FATS
10. Monounsaturated Fats
11. Polyunsaturated Fats
12. Saturated Fats

OTHERS LISTS
13. Free Foods
14. Combination Foods
15. Fast Foods

CARBOHYDRATE COUNTING

When you eat a healthy meal or snack, it is usually a mixture of carbohydrate, protein, and fat. However, your body changes carbohydrate into glucose faster than it changes protein and fat into glucose. It is the carbohydrate that makes your blood glucose level go up.

In carbohydrate counting, you count foods that are mostly carbohydrate. These include starches (breads, cereals, pasta), fruits and fruit juices, milk, yogurt, ice cream, and sugars (honey, syrup). You do not count most vegetables, meats, or fats. These foods have very little carbohydrate in them.

You can find out how much carbohydrate a food has by looking at the *Exchange Lists for Meal Planning, Basic Carbohydrate Counting*, the Nutrition Facts on food labels (see Food Labeling), or by asking your dietitian.

Knowing how much carbohydrate a food has can help you control your blood glucose levels. If you take at least three or four doses of insulin a day or use an insulin pump, you can learn to adjust each insulin dose to cover the amount of carbohydrate you eat. If you do not take insulin, you can learn how to space carbohydrate throughout the day to improve your blood glucose levels.

FOOD PYRAMID

For years, the guide to healthy eating had been the Basic Four Food Groups. But in 1992, the U.S. Department of Agriculture (USDA) changed the four food groups into six food groups. And they put the six food groups into sections of a pyramid. They called it the Food Guide Pyramid.

In 1995, The American Dietetic Association and the American Diabetes Association adapted the USDA Food Guide Pyramid into a pyramid just for people with diabetes. It is called the Diabetes Food Pyramid (see next page).

Your dietitian can help you learn how to divide the recommended number of servings noted on the pyramid into the meals and snacks you eat in a day. When using the pyramid, keep these three things in mind:

Variety. Eat a wide variety of foods from the food groups to get all the nutrients you need. For instance, eat more than one kind of vegetable.

Balance. Eat larger amounts and more servings from food groups that take up more space on the pyramid. The three food groups that take up more space are 1) grains, beans, and starchy vegetables; 2) vegetables; and 3) fruits.

Eat smaller amounts and fewer servings from food groups that take up less space on the pyramid. The three food groups that take up less space are 1) milk; 2) meat and others; and 3) fats, sweets, and alcohol.

Moderation. Eat the right amount of food. How much you eat depends on your health goals, calorie and nutrition needs, activity level, and

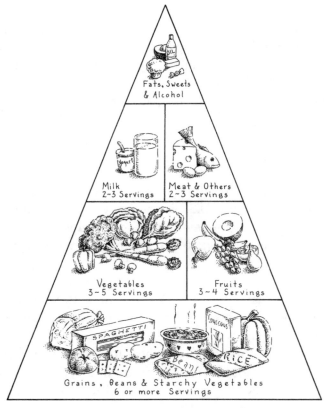

Diabetes Food Pyramid

insulin or diabetes pills. Your dietitian can help you figure out how much to eat.

For more information about using the Diabetes Food Pyramid as a meal-planning tool, see *Diabetes Meal Planning Made Easy: How to Put the Food Pyramid to Work for Your Busy Lifestyle*, 2nd Ed., by Hope Warshaw, MMSc, RD, CDE.

WHEN TO SEE YOUR DIETITIAN

See your dietitian regularly when you are first learning to use your meal-planning tool. Then review your meal plan with your dietitian every 6 months to a year. Ask your dietitian about other meal-planning tools.

Nerve Damage

Nerve damage is called neuropathy. Neuropathy affects the nerves outside your brain and spinal cord. These are called peripheral nerves. There are three types of peripheral nerves: motor, sensory, and autonomic. Neuropathy can affect any of these nerves.

Motor nerves control your voluntary movement. Voluntary movements are those you make yourself do, such as sitting, standing, and walking. Damage to the motor nerves can make your muscles weak and not able to do these things.

Sensory nerves allow you to feel and touch. Sensory nerves tell you if something is hot or cold. With sensory nerves, you can feel whether something is smooth or rough, soft or hard. Sensory nerves also let you feel pain. Damage to the sensory nerves can cause a loss of feeling.

Autonomic nerves control involuntary activities. Involuntary activities are those your body does without you having to tell it to. You do not have to tell your lungs to breathe in and out or your heart to beat. You do not have to tell your stomach to digest food. Damage to the autonomic nerves can make it hard for your body's organs to work.

There are many types of neuropathy. Two of the most common are distal symmetric polyneuropathy and autonomic neuropathy.

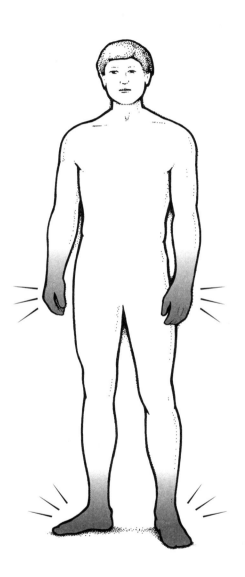

Distal symmetric polyneuropathy can
affect your feet, legs, or hands.

DISTAL SYMMETRIC POLYNEUROPATHY

Distal symmetric polyneuropathy is nerve damage to the feet and legs and sometimes to the hands. Distal means it affects parts of the body that are far from the trunk. Symmetric means it occurs on both sides of the body. Polyneuropathy means that more than one nerve is damaged.

Signs of nerve damage to the feet, legs, or hands

- Coldness, numbness
- Tingling, burning
- Itching, prickling
- Sensation of bugs crawling over your skin
- Sensation of walking on a strange surface
- Muscle weakness
- Deep aching
- Overly sensitive skin
- Pain on contact with sheets or clothing
- Electric shock–like sensations
- Jabs of needle-like pain

If you feel any of these signs, tell your doctor. The signs of nerve damage to the feet, legs, or hands tend to be worse at night. Signs often get better if you get out of bed and walk around a bit.

AUTONOMIC NEUROPATHY

Your autonomic nerves control your heart, lungs, blood vessels, stomach, intestines, bladder, and sex organs.

Heart, lungs, and blood vessels

Nerve damage to your heart, lungs, and blood vessels can affect your heart rate and blood pressure. Your heart may pound hard and fast when you are at rest. You may get dizzy or feel faint when you stand up quickly. Your blood pressure may go up when you are sleeping and down when you are standing. You may have a painless heart attack.

Stomach, intestines, and bladder

Nerve damage to your stomach can affect digestion. You may feel bloated, even after a small meal, and sick to your stomach. You may vomit food that you ate more than one meal before.

Damage to nerves in your intestines can cause diarrhea or constipation. If the nerves in your bladder are damaged, you will not be able to tell when your bladder is full of urine. You may dribble or wet yourself. The urine that stays in your bladder may cause a urinary tract infection.

Signs of a urinary tract infection include the need to urinate often, pain or burning when you urinate, cloudy or bloody urine, low back pain or abdominal pain, fever, and chills.

Sex organs

Nerve damage to the sex organs can cause impotence in men and vaginal dryness or loss of sensation in women (see Sex and Diabetes).

HOW TO PREVENT OR LESSEN NERVE DAMAGE

Keep blood glucose levels close to normal. When you have too much glucose in your blood, a lot of it goes into your nerve cells. Once inside nerve cells, this excess glucose forms sugar alcohols. The sugar alcohols build up, and your nerve cells don't work as well. After years of too much glucose, the nerves become damaged.

Stop smoking. Your nerves are fed by small blood vessels. Smoking damages these small blood vessels. Damaged blood vessels don't get oxygen to your nerves. Nerves without oxygen get damaged. If you already have nerve damage, smoking will make it worse.

Drink less alcohol. Drinking too much alcohol may cause nerve damage. If you already have nerve damage, drinking alcohol will make it worse.

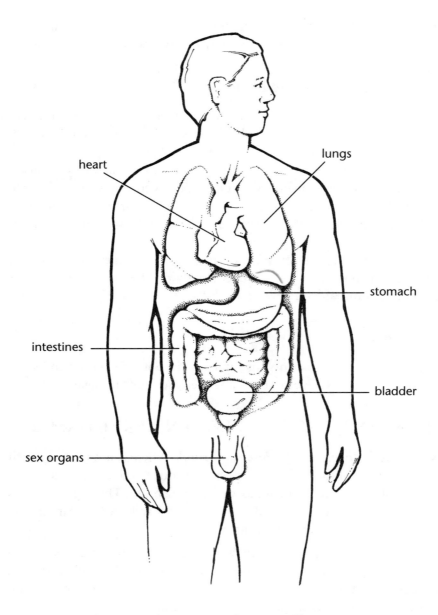

Autonomic neuropathy can affect your
heart, lungs, blood vessels, stomach, intestines,
bladder, or sex organs.

Keep blood pressure under 130/80 mmHg. High blood pressure is hard on your blood vessels. Weakened blood vessels don't nourish your nerves as well. The nerves get damaged.

Keep cholesterol levels under 200 mg/dl. High cholesterol can damage your blood vessels. Damaged blood vessels can't give your nerves the oxygen they need. Your nerves get damaged.

Have a yearly check for nerve damage. A doctor can do several different tests to find out how your nerves are doing. If damage is found, you can get treatments. The earlier damage is detected, the better the response to treatment.

Nutrition

Nutrition means getting nutrients—protein, carbohydrates, fats, vitamins, and minerals—from what you eat and drink. What you eat and drink will affect your blood glucose level and your weight.

The American Diabetes Association (ADA) sets nutrition guidelines for people with diabetes. Many of these guidelines are the same for people without diabetes.

CALORIES

The ADA recommends that you and your health care team decide how many calories you need to eat in a day to stay at a healthy weight.

Remember, fat has more than twice as many calories as carbohydrate or protein. One gram of carbohydrate has 4 calories. One gram of protein also has 4 calories. One gram of fat has 9 calories.

CARBOHYDRATE

The ADA recommends that you and your health care team decide exactly how much carbohydrate you will eat in a day. Carbohydrate includes both sugars and starches (see Healthy Eating).

CHOLESTEROL

The ADA recommends that you eat less than 300 milligrams of cholesterol per day. If you have high LDL cholesterol levels, eat less than 200 milligrams per day.

FAT

If your blood fat levels are normal and you are not overweight

Get less than 30 percent of calories from fat.

Get less than 10 percent of calories from saturated fat.

If you have high LDL cholesterol levels

Get less than 30 percent of calories from fat.

Get less than 7 percent of calories from saturated fat.

If you are overweight

Get 20 to 25 percent of calories from fat.

FIBER

The ADA recommends that you get 20 to 35 grams of fiber per day. This recommendation is the same whether you have diabetes or not.

PROTEIN

The ADA recommends that you get 10 to 20 percent of your daily calories from protein. If you have kidney disease, the ADA recommends that you get about 10 percent of your daily calories from protein.

SODIUM

One general rule is to get no more than 1 milligram of sodium for each calorie you eat in a day. For example, if you are on a 2,000-calorie diet, you would get no more than 2,000 milligrams of sodium each day. The ADA recommends that:

If you have normal blood pressure

Get no more than 2,400 milligrams of sodium per day.

If you have mild to moderately high blood pressure

Get less than 2,400 milligrams of sodium per day.

If you have high blood pressure and kidney disease

Get 1,500 milligrams or less of sodium per day.

SUGAR SUBSTITUTES

The ADA approves the use of four sugar substitutes in moderate amounts. These are aspartame (Nutrasweet, Equal), saccharin (Sweet'n Low, Sprinkle Sweet, Sweet-10, Sugar Twin), acesulfame potassium (Sweet One, Sunette), and sucralose (Splenda).

The U.S. Food and Drug Administration (FDA) establishes Acceptable Daily Intakes (ADIs) for sugar substitutes. These are the estimated amounts, based on body weight, that a person can safely consume every day over a lifetime.

	Acceptable Daily Intake (mg/kg body weight)	One Packet of Tabletop Sweetener (mg)
Acesulfame K	15	50
Aspartame	50	37
Saccharin	5	40
Sucralose	5–15	5

Oral Diabetes Medications

Right now, oral diabetes medications consist of diabetes pills that help people with type 2 diabetes control blood glucose levels. They are not insulin. (However, new types of oral medications, such as insulin that can be inhaled or taken orally, may soon be available.) Doctors may prescribe diabetes pills for people who are not able to keep their blood glucose at safe levels with healthy eating and exercise.

There are now five classes of diabetes pills available in the United States: sulfonylureas, biguanides, alpha-glucosidase inhibitors, thiazolidinediones, and meglitinides.

SULFONYLUREAS

The first class of diabetes pills is the sulfonylureas. Newer drugs in this class include glimepiride (Amaryl), glipizide (Glucotrol and Glucotrol XL), and glyburide (Diabeta, Glynase PresTab, Micronase).

Sulfonylureas help your body send out more of its own insulin. They may help your body respond to insulin. And they may stop your liver from putting stored glucose into your blood. These actions lower your blood glucose.

Possible side effects of sulfonylureas

- Gastrointestinal trouble:
    constipation, diarrhea, cramping, heartburn, stomach fullness, lack of appetite, nausea, vomiting
- Low blood glucose reaction (see Blood Glucose, Low)

- Skin reaction:
    itching, hives, rash, sun sensitivity
- Weight gain

Alert your doctor to any possible side effects you notice after you start taking sulfonylureas. Do not take sulfonylureas if you are pregnant, have allergies to sulfa drugs, or have liver or kidney disease.

BIGUANIDES

The second class of diabetes pills is the biguanides. Metformin (Glucophage) is the only biguanide currently available in the United States. Biguanides cause your liver to release stored glucose more slowly. They may also help your body respond to insulin. These actions keep your blood glucose levels more even.

Possible side effects of biguanides

- Nausea
- Bloating
- Cramping
- Diarrhea
- Loss of appetite

These side effects can be minimized by starting with a low dose and by taking the drug with food. Biguanides can cause lactic acidosis in people with heart, kidney, or liver disease, or in those who have taken an X-ray dye test. Lactic acidosis is a life-threatening buildup of acid in the blood. Do not take biguanides if you have heart, kidney, or liver disease, or when you are having an X-ray dye test.

ALPHA-GLUCOSIDASE INHIBITORS

The third class of diabetes pills is the alpha-glucosidase inhibitors. The two currently available drugs in this class are acarbose (Precose) and glyset (Miglitol).

Alpha-glucosidase inhibitors slow the time it takes for your intestine to break down some carbohydrates into glucose. This causes glucose to enter your blood more slowly. Your blood glucose level then stays more even, with fewer highs and lows. Acarbose is especially helpful at flattening out the sharp rise in glucose that may occur after meals.

Possible side effects of alpha-glucosidase inhibitors

- Gas
- Bloating
- Diarrhea

These side effects can be minimized by starting with a low dose. Do not take alpha-glucosidase inhibitors if you have any gastrointestinal diseases.

THIAZOLIDINEDIONES

The fourth class of diabetes pills is the thiazolidinediones. This class includes pioglitazone hydrochloride (Actos) and rosiglitazone (Avandia). These drugs make your muscle cells more sensitive to insulin. They may also reduce the release of stored glucose by the liver.

Possible side effects of thiazolidinediones

- Weight gain
- Edema
- Congestive heart failure

Thiazolidinediones can cause liver damage. Because of this, the U.S. Food and Drug Administration (FDA) recommends a liver test before starting any of them. During the first year of therapy, the FDA recommends a liver test every 2 months for people taking either Avandia or Actos. After that, the FDA advises periodic testing for those using either Avandia or Actos.

Signs of liver damage

- Nausea
- Vomiting
- Abdominal pain
- Fatigue
- Loss of appetite
- Dark urine
- Jaundice

Call your doctor right away if you have any of the signs of liver damage. Do not use thiazolidinediones if you are pregnant, have liver disease, or have congestive heart failure.

MEGLITINIDES

The fifth class of diabetes pills is the meglitinides. Repaglinide (Prandin) is the only meglitinide currently available in the United States. Like the sulfonylureas, meglitinides help your body send out more of its own insulin. This lowers your blood glucose. Unlike the sulfonylureas, meglitinides work very quickly and are meant to be taken just before meals. This keeps glucose levels from rising too high after meals.

Possible side effects of meglitinides

- Low blood glucose reaction
- Headache
- Nausea
- Upper respiratory tract infection
- Nasal and sinus inflammation
- Bronchitis
- Back pain
- Joint pain
- Weight gain

You can reduce the risk of low blood glucose if you always take the drug with food.

PART OF A DIABETES CARE PLAN

Diabetes pills do not take the place of healthy eating and exercise. They work with healthy eating and exercise. In fact, if you do not follow your meal and exercise plans, diabetes pills may not work for you.

Sometimes, diabetes pills work for a little while, then stop working. This often happens after several years. If your pills stop working, then your doctor may put you on another pill, two or three different types of pills, a pill and insulin, or insulin alone.

You and your health care team will need to work together to find the best treatment for you.

Pre-Diabetes

Pre-diabetes is a condition where blood glucose levels are higher than normal, but not high enough to be diagnosed as diabetes. Generally, a person with pre-diabetes has either impaired fasting glucose (IFG) or impaired glucose tolerance (IGT). Although pre-diabetes is not a type of diabetes, if you have it, you are more likely to get diabetes. Doctors might call pre-diabetes by other names, such as:

- A touch of sugar
- Borderline diabetes
- Chemical diabetes
- Latent diabetes
- Potential diabetes
- Subclinical diabetes

Many people with pre-diabetes show no signs of illness and may have normal or near-normal A1C levels (see A1C Test). The only way to know for sure whether you have pre-diabetes is through the following blood tests done by your doctor.

FASTING BLOOD GLUCOSE TEST

This test is used to determine whether or not you have IFG, a component of pre-diabetes. In the fasting blood glucose test, your blood glucose level is measured when you have not eaten for 8 to 12 hours. That is why it is usually done first thing in the morning.

A person without diabetes has a fasting blood glucose level below 100 mg/dl. A person with diabetes has a fasting blood glucose level of 126 mg/dl or above. A person with IFG has a fasting blood glucose level between 100 and 126 mg/dl.

ORAL GLUCOSE TOLERANCE TEST

This test is used to determine whether or not you have IGT, another form of pre-diabetes. In the oral glucose tolerance test, your blood glucose levels are measured at fasting and then 2 hours after the test. First, your blood glucose is measured when you have not eaten for 8 to 12 hours (same as the fasting blood glucose test).

Then you drink a liquid with 75 grams of glucose in it (100 grams for pregnant women). Your blood glucose is then measured at 2 hours after the drink.

In a person without diabetes, the blood glucose level is below 140 mg/dl at 2 hours after the drink. In a person with diabetes, the blood glucose level is 200 mg/dl or above at 2 hours after the drink. In a person with IGT, the blood glucose level is between 140 and 200 mg/dl at 2 hours after the drink.

WHAT TO DO IF YOU HAVE PRE-DIABETES

If you have pre-diabetes, you are more likely to be overweight, to have high triglyceride levels, to have low HDL levels, and to have high blood pressure. These put you at increased risk for heart disease.

If you have pre-diabetes, go back to your doctor at least once a year to have your blood glucose tested. In the meantime, there are a few things you can do to return your blood glucose levels to normal and decrease your other risk factors:

- Lose weight (if you are overweight).
- Lower your triglyceride and LDL cholesterol levels (if they are high).
- Lower your blood pressure (if it is high).
- Exercise or increase your activity.
- Eat healthy foods.

Pregnancy

Most women with diabetes have healthy babies. Often the biggest fear of women with diabetes is that their baby will get diabetes. In fact, the chances that their baby will get diabetes are small.

THE CHANCES THAT A BABY WILL GET DIABETES

If the mother has type 1 diabetes

The baby has a 1 to 3 percent chance of getting type 1 diabetes.

If the father has type 1 diabetes

The baby has a 3 to 6 percent chance of getting type 1 diabetes.

If either parent gets type 2 diabetes after age 50

The baby has a 7 percent chance of getting diabetes.

If either parent gets type 2 diabetes before age 50

The baby has a 14 percent chance of getting diabetes.

Although your baby may be safe from diabetes, there are other potential dangers to your baby's health and your own.

HIGH BLOOD GLUCOSE

One of the biggest dangers to you and your baby is high blood glucose levels. High blood glucose levels can lead to birth defects, macrosomia (see below), and low blood glucose in your baby and to urinary tract infections in you.

Birth defects. High blood glucose levels during the first 8 weeks of your pregnancy can cause birth defects. It is during these early weeks that your baby's organs are forming.

Birth defects can affect any part of your baby. The heart, spinal cord, brain, and bones are most often affected. Because you have diabetes, birth defects are more likely to be severe and to cause miscarriages.

Macrosomia. Macrosomia means large body. If your blood glucose is too high during pregnancy, your baby may grow bigger and fatter than normal. This makes delivery harder. Babies who are larger than normal are more likely to have health problems.

Low blood glucose. High blood glucose levels right before or during labor can cause your baby to have low blood glucose after delivery.

Urinary tract infections. When your blood glucose is high during pregnancy, you are more likely to get a urinary tract infection. Urinary tract infections are usually caused by bacteria. Bacteria grow much better and faster in high glucose.

Signs of a urinary tract infection include the need to urinate often, pain or burning when you urinate, cloudy or bloody urine, low back pain or abdominal pain, fever, and chills.

HIGH KETONES

Ketones are made when your body burns stored fat for energy. Large amounts of ketones can harm you or your baby. Ketones are more likely to build up if you are not eating and drinking enough for both you and your baby. Be sure to eat all meals and snacks at your scheduled times.

DIABETES PILLS

Diabetes pills are not used during pregnancy because they may cause birth defects and low blood glucose in your baby. If you take diabetes pills, stop taking them before you get pregnant and while you are pregnant.

Your doctor may need to switch you to insulin. You may need insulin from early on in your pregnancy or just at the end of your pregnancy. Or you may not need any insulin at all.

PREECLAMPSIA

Preeclampsia (also called toxemia) is high blood pressure, swelling of your feet and lower legs, and leaking of protein into your urine during pregnancy. Other signs include headache, nausea, vomiting, abdominal pain, and blurred sight. If not treated, preeclampsia can cause seizures, coma, and death to you or your baby. Your doctor will watch for signs of preeclampsia.

HYDRAMNIOS

Hydramnios is excess amniotic fluid in your uterus. Signs of hydramnios are abdominal discomfort, larger-than-usual uterus, shortness of breath, and swelling of your legs. Hydramnios may cause premature labor. Your doctor will watch for signs of hydramnios.

HOW TO ENSURE YOUR BABY'S HEALTH

Get your blood glucose in good control before pregnancy. If your blood glucose is in poor control, try to bring it into good control 3 to 6 months before you plan to get pregnant. If you wait until you know you are pregnant, your baby could already be harmed.

Keep your blood glucose in good control during your pregnancy. This will require more frequent blood glucose checking—sometimes up to eight times a day. Staying in good control will reduce the risk of problems for both you and your baby. It will also make it easier for you and your health care team to adjust your insulin dosage and/or meal plan.

Check your urine for ketones every morning. If you have moderate to large amounts of ketones in your urine, contact your doctor right away. You may need a change in your meal plan or insulin.

Get fit before you get pregnant. Exercising before pregnancy may increase your endurance, help lower your blood glucose, help you lose weight, and build strength and flexibility.

Exercise during your pregnancy. Pregnancy is not the time to start a vigorous exercise program, but you will most likely be able to continue an exercise you were doing regularly before pregnancy. If you were not exercising regularly before pregnancy, ask your doctor about exercises that would be safe for you and your baby. Some good exercises for pregnant women include walking, low-impact aerobics, swimming, and water aerobics.

Follow your pregnancy meal plan. A pregnancy meal plan is designed to help you avoid high and low blood glucose while providing what your baby needs to grow. Three meals and three snacks a day are often the rule. Occasionally, a middle-of-the-night snack may be necessary. It may even be necessary to meet with your dietitian every 3 months or so during the pregnancy to update the meal plan based on the changing needs of your body and the baby.

Quit Smoking

Quitting smoking is good for your diabetes. Quitting smoking is good for your health. When you quit smoking, you lower your blood glucose and blood pressure. You lower your total cholesterol, LDL cholesterol (the bad kind), and your triglycerides. When you quit smoking, you raise your HDL cholesterol (the good kind) and your oxygen intake. You even raise your life expectancy!

Quit smoking and you can reduce your risk for heart disease, blood vessel damage, kidney disease, nerve damage, dental disease, and cancer (mouth, throat, lungs, and bladder). You can reduce your risk of heart attack and stroke, miscarriage or stillbirth, limited joint mobility, and colds, bronchitis, and emphysema.

Quit smoking and you can even reduce your risk for insulin resistance (when your body does not respond to insulin). No wonder people try to quit. Here are some helpful hints.

BEFORE YOU QUIT SMOKING

Write down each time you smoke for a week. Write down any event or activity you were doing or about to do. Save the list.

Write down all the reasons you want to quit. Read the list each day of the week before you quit.

Pick a day to quit and write it down. Choose a day with few pressures. That way, stress won't tempt you to smoke. You may want to do it when you've got some time off from work.

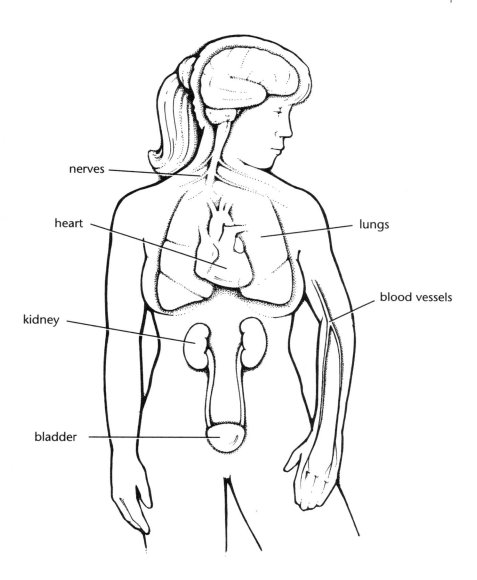

Smoking can damage your heart, lungs, blood vessels, nerves, kidneys, and bladder. Smoking increases your risk of heart attack, stroke, miscarriages, and stillbirths.

Tell others you plan to quit. Let family, friends, and coworkers know. Seek their support. Tell them how they can help you. For example, ask them not to offer you a cigarette. Tell them what to expect when you first quit (see below).

Choose a method of quitting. There are many ways to quit smoking. Not every method works for every person. Your diabetes care team may be able to help you find a method that will work for you. It could be quitting "cold turkey." It might be using a nicotine patch or chewing gum. Hypnosis helps some people stop smoking. For others, acupuncture stops the craving to smoke.

Consider joining a stop-smoking class. You may find it easier to quit with other people. Check for classes at local hospitals or local branches of organizations, such as the American Lung Association, the American Heart Association, and the American Cancer Society.

Practice deep breathing. Relaxation tapes may help.

Stock up on low-fat, low-calorie snacks. Your appetite may increase after you quit smoking. You may gain weight (the average gain is 7 pounds). You may crave sweet foods.

Begin to exercise a few weeks before you quit smoking. More activity will help you combat withdrawal symptoms and weight gain. Exercise can take the place of smoking or help you control the urge to eat. Try brisk walking, cycling, or swimming.

Plan rewards for not smoking. For example, you might play a favorite game one week, and go to a movie the next week.

WHEN YOU QUIT SMOKING

You may go through withdrawal for a few days or weeks. The table on the next page lists some of the symptoms you may feel and how to deal with them.

AFTER YOU QUIT SMOKING

The first 3 months or so after quitting are the hardest. Most people who return to smoking do so then. Try these tactics for staying smoke-free.

WITHDRAWAL

Symptom	Duration	Solution
Urge to smoke	Strong first 2 weeks, then on and off	Do something else.
Blood glucose goes up and down	Varies	Monitor closely.
Irritable, tense, on edge	Several weeks	Take a break or a walk. Listen to a relaxation tape.
Trouble concentrating or feel "out of it"	Several weeks	Break up big tasks into smaller ones. Take short breaks.
Extra energy or restlessness	Varies	Exercise.
Sleepy during the day	2 to 4 weeks	Take a walk or a nap.
Trouble sleeping at night	Less than 7 days	Try deep breathing. Avoid caffeine after 5 P.M.
Constipation	3 to 4 weeks	Add fiber (fresh fruits, vegetables, whole-grain breads and cereals) to meal plan. Drink 6 to 8 glasses of water a day.
Coughing	Less than 7 days	Sip water.
Headache, muscle cramps, nausea, or sweating	Few days	Try a warm bath or some quiet time.
Craving sweets	Several weeks	Eat a low-calorie snack.

- Refer to the list you made of events or activities that were going on around the time you smoked. The next time any of those events or activities come up, avoid them. For example, if you always smoke at happy hour, don't go. If you can't avoid the event, replace the cigarette with something else. Hold something else in your hand. Try a strand of beads, a polished stone, or a pen. Put something else in your mouth, like a toothpick. Chew gum or ice.
- If you smoke to relax, find another way to relax. Try deep breathing or relaxation exercises. If you smoke to perk up, try a walk or stretching.
- Throw away your cigarettes, butts, lighters, matches, and ashtrays.
- Put your list of reasons for quitting where you had kept your cigarettes.
- Read your list of reasons for quitting. Remind yourself that you don't want to smoke.
- Remind yourself that all it takes is one cigarette to become a smoker again. Try to avoid even one.
- Make a list of things you like about not smoking.
- If you are worried about gaining weight, talk with your dietitian about changing your meal and exercise plans.

Relieve Stress

Our lives are full of things that can cause stress. Traffic jams, holiday travel, unemployment, divorce, or an illness, such as diabetes, can all cause stress. Working to relieve this stress can have a dramatic impact on your diabetes care and your well-being.

WHAT CAUSES YOU TO FEEL STRESSED?

Each one of us is different. What causes little or no stress for you may cause great stress for somebody else. Make a list of the people or things that stress you.

WHAT HAPPENS TO YOUR BODY WHEN YOU ARE STRESSED?

When you feel stressed, your body gets ready for action. It pumps stress hormones into your blood. Stress hormones make your body release stored glucose and stored fat for extra energy. This extra energy helps your body face up to or run away from the stress. But the extra glucose and fat can only be used by your body if there is enough insulin.

In people with diabetes, there may not be enough insulin. And the stress hormones themselves may make it harder for your body to use the insulin that is there. When there is not enough insulin, glucose and fat build up in the blood. This can lead to high glucose levels and high ketones. To avoid high glucose and high ketones, you need to know what happens to your blood glucose level when you are under stress.

WHAT HAPPENS TO YOUR BLOOD GLUCOSE LEVEL WHEN YOU ARE STRESSED?

The type of stress you are under may make a difference. Physical stress, such as an injury or an illness, causes blood glucose levels to go up in most people with diabetes. Mental stress, such as problems with your marriage or finances, causes some people's glucose levels to go up and other people's glucose levels to go down. To see which way your blood glucose level goes, try the following test.

Blood glucose stress test

Before you check your blood glucose, rate your level of stress. You can use a number from 1 to 10 or the words *high*, *medium*, or *low*. Write down your stress rating. Now check your blood glucose. Record your results. Do this for a week or two.

Compare the blood glucose results with your stress ratings. Does high blood glucose occur with high stress? If so, you may need more insulin when you are under stress. Check with your diabetes care provider first.

HOW DO YOU REACT TO STRESS?

Pay attention to how you react. How you react may be different from how someone else reacts. You may react by feeling tense, anxious, upset, or angry. You may react by feeling tired, sad, or empty. Your stomach, head, or back may hurt.

Some people react by laughing nervously or being self-critical. Others become easily discouraged or frustrated or bored. Some cry easily.

HOW DO YOU HANDLE STRESS?

How you handle each stressful situation determines how much stress you feel. You can handle stress in a way that makes you feel in control. Or you can handle stress in a way that makes you feel worse.

Some people choose to handle stress in ways that are damaging. They may turn to alcohol, caffeine, nicotine, or anything they think might lift or calm them. Some choose to binge on food.

Any excessive behavior, even gambling or oversleeping, may be a way to try to get away from stress. These solutions seldom work, and with diabetes, most of them are dangerous. There are other, safer stress relievers.

HOW TO HANDLE STRESS SAFELY

Breathe deeply. Sit or lie down. Uncross your legs and arms. Close your eyes. Breathe in deeply and slowly. Let all the breath out. Breathe in and out again. Start to relax your muscles. Keep breathing in and out. Each time you breathe out, relax your muscles even more. Do this for 5 to 20 minutes. Do it at least once a day.

Let go. Lie down. Close your eyes. Tense, hold, and then release the muscles of each body part. Start at your head and work your way down to your feet.

Loosen up. Circle, stretch, and shake parts of your body.

Stay active. Some of the best activities for relieving stress are cross training, cross-country skiing, bicycling, rowing, running, and swimming. If you don't like any of these, find another activity you like and do it often.

Get a massage. Put yourself in the hands of a licensed massage therapist.

Think good thoughts. Your thoughts affect your feelings. Put a rubber band on your wrist. Snap it each time you think a bad thought. Replace that bad thought with a better thought. Or repeat a happy poem, prayer, or quote that calms and focuses you.

Talk about it. Find someone to talk to when something is bothering you. It may make you feel better. Confide in family or friends. Consult a therapist or join a support group. Others may be having the same troubles you are.

Put it on paper. Write down what's bothering you. You may find a solution. Or draw or paint your worries away.

Try something new. Start a hobby or learn a craft. Take a class. Join a club or a team. Volunteer to help others. Form a discussion group on books, movies, or whatever interests you. Start a potluck dinner group.

Get away. Go on a minivacation or overnighter. Take a long weekend. Form a baby-sitting cooperative with other parents so you can get out more.

Listen up. Listen to music you find soothing. Or play a tape of nature sounds, such as birds or ocean waves.

Soak in a warm bath. The most comfortable bath water is about the same temperature as your skin—probably between 85° and 93° F. Linger in the bath for 20 to 30 minutes. Add bubbles or soothing herbs if you like.

Say "no." Especially to things you really don't want to do. You may feel stressed if you take on too much.

Laugh about it. Have a hearty, healthy laugh every day. Seek out funny movies, funny books, and funny people.

Look at nature. Look at the world around you. Flowers, trees, even bugs. The sun, the moon, the stars. Clouds, wind, and rain. Just go outside and spend time there. If you can't go outside, look out a window. Even looking at pictures of nature can help you slow down and relax.

Eat wisely. When you are under stress, your body may use up more B vitamins, vitamin C, protein, and calcium. Replenish your B vitamins by eating more whole grains, nuts, seeds, and beans. Boost your vitamin C with oranges, grapefruits, and broccoli. Beef up your protein with chicken, fish, and egg whites. Stock up your calcium with low-fat milk, yogurt, and cheese.

Sleep on it. Sometimes things look better the next day. Get your daily 7 to 9 hours of sleep.

Sex and Diabetes

Diabetes and its complications can hurt your sex life. Sexual problems may have both physical and psychological causes. Doctors usually look for physical causes of sexual problems first.

PHYSICAL CAUSES

Too tired. If your blood glucose levels are high, you may feel too tired to have sex. Getting your diabetes under better control can help.

Urinary tract infection. When your blood glucose level is high, you are more likely to get a urinary tract infection. Signs of a urinary tract infection include:

- Frequent urination
- Pain or burning during urination
- Cloudy or bloody urine
- Low back pain or abdominal pain
- Fever
- Chills

Sex may be painful or uncomfortable if you have a urinary tract infection. Urinary tract infections can be treated with antibiotic drugs.

Lack of bladder control. If you have nerve damage to your bladder, you will not be able to tell when your bladder is full of urine. You may dribble or wet yourself during sex or orgasm. To prevent this, try emptying your bladder before and after sex.

Damaged limbs or joints. If you have nerve damage to a limb, are missing a limb, or have a joint disease, sex may be awkward or uncomfortable. Try different positions. Some may be better than others. Supporting yourself with several pillows may help. A physical therapist may be able to suggest ways for you to be more comfortable during sex.

Women only

Loss of sensation. Nerve damage to the sex organs can cause a loss of sensation. This can make it harder for a woman to reach orgasm. Kegel exercises, changes in position during sex, and more intense direct stimulation of the sex organs may help.

Vaginal infection (vaginitis). Women with diabetes tend to get more vaginal infections than women without diabetes. Most vaginal infections are caused by the fungus *Candida albicans*. High blood glucose levels encourage the fungus to grow. Signs of vaginitis include:

- Thick white discharge
- Itching
- Burning
- Redness
- Swelling

Vaginitis can cause irritation, discomfort, or pain during or after sex. Antifungal creams or drugs can clear up most vaginal infections. Getting your blood glucose under control may help prevent them.

Vaginal dryness. Nerve damage to the cells that line your vagina can cause vaginal dryness. Vaginal dryness can cause irritation, discomfort, or pain during or after sex. Over-the-counter or prescription lubricants can help. Getting your blood glucose under control may delay or slow nerve damage.

Vaginal tightness (vaginismus). The pain or discomfort that you feel from vaginal infections or vaginal dryness can make you more likely to have vaginismus. Vaginismus is an involuntary spasm of the muscles around the vaginal entrance. It can make sex difficult or painful. Learning to relax these muscles through Kegel exercises can help. Trying positions in which you have more control over penetration can also help.

Men only

Impotence. About half of men with diabetes become impotent. Impotence means that the penis does not become or stay hard enough for sex. There are many causes of impotence. The most common causes of impotence in men with diabetes are:

- Damage to the nerves in your penis
- Damage to the blood vessels in your penis
- Poor control over your blood glucose levels

Physical impotence usually happens slowly and gets worse. Signs include a less rigid penis and fewer erections. Eventually, there are no erections. Keeping your blood glucose levels under control is the best way to avoid impotence. If you do become impotent, talk with your doctor. There are many treatment choices for physical impotence.

PSYCHOLOGICAL CAUSES

If you and your doctor have not been able to find a physical cause for your sexual problem, there may be a psychological cause. Psychological causes of sexual problems are the same whether you have diabetes or not. A sexual problem may be psychological if:

- You are not able to talk with your partner about sex.
- You and your partner argue over money, children, or work.
- You are stressed, worried, or anxious.
- You fear impotence.
- You fear pregnancy.
- You are sad, depressed, or angry.
- You had an inadequate sex education.

- You had a restrictive upbringing.
- You have been sexually abused.

If you think a psychological cause is a part of your sexual problem, seek out a mental health professional who specializes in this area. This might be a psychiatrist, psychologist, or licensed social worker.

Sick Days

Being sick with a cold or the flu can upset your diabetes care plan. You may not be able to eat as you usually do or take your usual diabetes pills or insulin. When you are sick, your blood glucose levels may go up too high or down too low.

Your health care team can help you make a sick-day plan before you get sick. Your sick-day plan will include what medicines to take, what to eat and drink, how often to check your blood glucose, when to call your diabetes care provider, and what to tell him or her.

WHAT MEDICINES TO TAKE

Only your diabetes care provider can tell you for sure what medicines to take. But most likely, you'll keep taking your insulin or diabetes pills.

If you control your diabetes with insulin, you may need to adjust your usual doses. If you control your diabetes with healthy eating and exercise or with diabetes pills, your health care provider may want you to take insulin when you are sick.

You may decide to take other kinds of medicines to care for your sickness. Some of these medicines may raise your blood glucose level and others may lower it. Ask your doctor or pharmacist whether the medicines you plan to take will affect your blood glucose level.

WHAT TO EAT AND DRINK

Eat foods from your usual meal plan if you can. If you can't eat your usual foods, follow your sick-day meal plan. It will include foods that are easy on your stomach. You may want to set aside a small area of your cupboard for sick-day foods.

If you have a fever, are throwing up, or have diarrhea, you may lose too much fluid. Try to drink a cup of fluid each hour.

If your blood glucose level is above 250 mg/dl, drink sugar-free liquids, such as water, caffeine-free tea, sugar-free ginger ale, or broth (chicken, beef, or vegetable).

If your blood glucose level is below 250 mg/dl, drink liquids with about 15 grams of carbohydrate in them (see list of sick-day foods and fluids below).

SICK-DAY FOODS AND FLUIDS WITH ~15 g OF CARBOHYDRATE

6 saltine crackers	1/2 cup ice cream
5 vanilla wafers	1/2 cup cooked cereal
3 graham crackers	1/2 cup mashed potatoes
1 fruit juice bar	1/3 cup cooked rice
1 slice toast or bread	3/4 cup plain yogurt
1 cup soup	1/3 cup frozen yogurt
1 cup low-fat milk	1/4 cup sherbet
1 cup sports drink	1/2 cup applesauce, unsweetened
1/3 cup fruit juice	1/4 cup pudding
1/2 cup regular gelatin	1/2 cup canned fruit

HOW OFTEN TO CHECK BLOOD GLUCOSE AND URINE KETONES

Usually, you will need to check your blood glucose and urine ketones more often when you are sick. The sick-day plan you work out with your health care team will tell you how often to check.

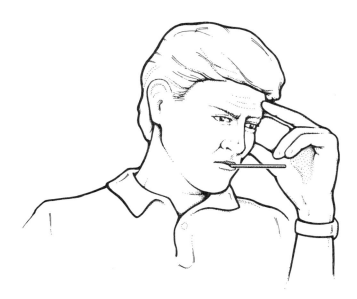

If you have type 1 diabetes, you may need to check your blood glucose and ketones every 3 to 4 hours. If you have type 2 diabetes, you may need to check your blood glucose four or five times a day.

WHEN TO CALL YOUR PROVIDER

Call your health care provider when:

- You have been sick for 2 days and you are not getting better.
- You have been throwing up or have had diarrhea for more than 6 hours.
- Your blood glucose level is staying above 250 mg/dl.
- Your blood glucose level is staying below 60 mg/dl.
- You have moderate or large amounts of ketones in your urine.
- You have any of these signs: chest pain, trouble breathing, fruity breath, or dry and cracked lips or tongue.
- You are not sure what to do to take care of yourself.

WHAT TO TELL YOUR PROVIDER

Keep written records so you can tell your diabetes care provider:

- How long you have been sick
- What medicines you have taken and how much
- Whether you have been able to eat and drink and how much
- Whether you are throwing up or have diarrhea
- Whether you have lost weight
- Your temperature
- Your blood glucose levels
- Your urine ketone levels

Know where to reach members of your health care team or their back-ups on weekends, holidays, and evenings. If you must talk to someone other than a member of your health care team, be sure to tell him or her about your diabetes.

HOW ABOUT EXERCISE?

Exercising when you are sick can make your blood glucose levels go down too low or up too high. If you exercise when you are sick, it may take longer for you to get better. You may even get bronchitis or pneumonia. Do not exercise when you are sick.

Find out from your diabetes care provider when it is safe to start exercising again. Because you may be less fit after being sick, ease into your exercise program. You might try exercising at a lower intensity, for a shorter time, or on fewer days.

Skin Care

Diabetes makes skin problems more likely. Some skin problems are ones that anyone can have but that people with diabetes get more easily. These include bacterial infections and fungal infections. Other skin problems happen mostly to people with diabetes. These include diabetic dermopathy and digital sclerosis.

BACTERIAL INFECTIONS

Three bacterial infections that people with diabetes get more easily than people without diabetes are sties, boils, and carbuncles. All three are most often caused by staphylococcal bacteria. All appear as red, painful, pus-filled lumps.

A sty is an infected gland of the eyelid. A boil is an infected hair root or skin gland. A carbuncle is a cluster of boils. Boils and carbuncles often occur at the back of your neck, armpits, groin, or buttocks.

If you think you have a sty, boil, carbuncle, or other bacterial infection, see your doctor.

FUNGAL INFECTIONS

Four fungal infections that people with diabetes get more easily than people without diabetes are jock itch, athlete's foot, ringworm, and vaginal infections.

Jock itch is a red, itchy area that spreads from your genitals outward over the inside of your thigh. In athlete's foot, the skin between your toes becomes itchy and sore. It may crack and peel, or blister.

Ringworm is a ring-shaped, red, scaly patch that may itch or blister. It can appear on your feet, groin, scalp, nails, or body.

Vaginal infections are often caused by the fungus *Candida albicans*. It causes a thick white discharge from your vagina and/or itching, burning, or irritation.

If you think you have a fungal infection, call your doctor.

DIABETIC DERMOPATHY

Some people with diabetes get a skin condition called diabetic dermopathy. It causes red or brown scaly patches to form, usually on the front of your legs. Diabetic dermopathy is harmless and needs no treatment.

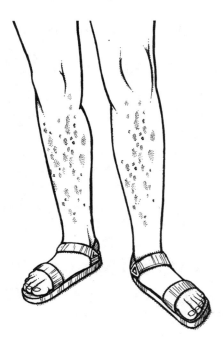

Diabetic dermopathy causes red or brown patches on the front of your legs.

DIGITAL SCLEROSIS

People with diabetes may also get digital sclerosis. Digital refers to your fingers or toes. Sclerosis means hardening.

Digital sclerosis causes the skin on your hands, fingers, or toes to become thick and tight and look waxy or shiny. It can also cause aching and stiffness in your fingers. It may even limit movement so that you cannot easily bring the palms of your hands together, as if praying.

There is no treatment for digital sclerosis. However, painkillers and anti-inflammatory drugs can relieve aching joints.

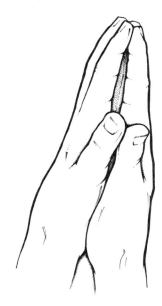

Digital sclerosis can make it hard to
press your palms together.

HOW TO CARE FOR YOUR SKIN

Keep your diabetes in good control. High blood glucose levels make it easier for you to get bacterial and fungal infections. High blood glucose levels also tend to give you dry skin.

Keep your skin clean. Take warm, not hot, baths or showers. Hot water can dry out your skin.

Keep dry parts of your skin moist. Use moisturizers and moisturizing soaps. Keep your home more humid during cold, dry months. Drink plenty of water. It helps keep your skin moist, too.

Keep other parts of your skin dry. Areas where skin touches skin need to be kept dry. These areas are between your toes, under your arms, and at your groin. Using powder on these areas can help keep them dry.

Protect your skin from the sun. The sun can dry and burn your skin. When you are out in the sun, wear a waterproof, sweatproof sunscreen with an SPF (sun protection factor) of at least 15. Wearing a hat also helps.

Treat minor skin problems. Over-the-counter products can be used to treat skin problems. But it's best to check with your diabetes care provider before using any skin treatment.

See a skin doctor. If you are prone to skin problems, ask your diabetes care provider about adding a skin doctor (dermatologist) to your health care team.

Stroke

A stroke occurs when blood flow to the brain is blocked. Without blood, the brain can't get the oxygen it needs. Part of the brain gets damaged or dies.

Blood flow can be cut off by a buildup of fat and cholesterol in the blood vessels that lead to the brain (atherosclerosis). This type of stroke is called an ischemic stroke. It is the most common type.

If blood flow to the brain is blocked for only a brief time, it is called a transient ischemic attack, or TIA. Your body may release enzymes that dissolve the clot quickly and restore blood flow. If you have TIAs often, you are more likely to have an ischemic stroke.

Another type of stroke is called a hemorrhagic stroke. It occurs when a blood vessel in your brain leaks or breaks. The most common cause of hemorrhagic strokes is high blood pressure. High blood pressure can weaken blood vessels. Weak blood vessels are more likely to leak or break.

Having diabetes doubles your chances of having a stroke. If you have other risk factors for stroke, your chances of having a stroke are even greater.

RISK FACTORS FOR STROKE

- You have had TIAs.
- You have high blood pressure.
- You smoke.
- You have high cholesterol.

- You are overweight.
- You do not exercise.
- You drink too much alcohol.

You can't change the fact that you have diabetes. But you can reduce your other risk factors.

HOW TO REDUCE YOUR RISK OF STROKE

Control your diabetes. Try to keep your blood glucose levels in your range (see Blood Glucose). This may prevent or delay blood vessel damage caused by high blood glucose.

Control high blood pressure. Work with your health care team to bring your blood pressure down with healthy eating, exercise, weight loss, and blood pressure drugs. Cutting down on sodium (salt) lowers blood pressure for some people.

Quit smoking. Smoking narrows blood vessels and promotes the buildup of fat and cholesterol on blood vessel walls. Smoking makes blood clot faster.

Eat less fat. Eating less saturated animal fats and cholesterol can lower your cholesterol level. High cholesterol can damage blood vessels.

Lose a few pounds! Losing even a little weight with healthy eating and more activity lowers blood pressure and improves cholesterol levels.

Get moving. Try walking or biking for as little as 15 minutes a day three times a week. These types of aerobic exercise can lower your blood pressure, lower your bad LDL cholesterol and triglycerides, and raise your good HDL cholesterol.

Cut back on alcohol. Drinking too much alcohol can raise your blood pressure. Men, drink no more than two drinks a day. Women, drink no more than one drink a day. A drink equals a 12 oz beer, 5 oz wine, or 1.5 oz liquor. Don't drink at all if you have a drinking problem or a medical reason not to drink.

Be alert to the warning signs of stroke. Know what to do if the warning signs occur.

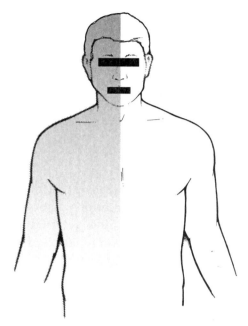

A stroke can cause difficulty seeing or talking or lead
to weakness on one side of your body.

WARNING SIGNS OF A STROKE OR TIA

- You are suddenly weak or numb in your face, an arm, or a leg.
- Your sight is suddenly dim, blurred, or lost.
- You can't speak or can't understand someone else who is talking.
- You have a sudden headache.
- You feel dizzy or unsteady, or you suddenly fall.

IF YOU THINK YOU ARE HAVING A STROKE

1. Call 911 for an ambulance.
2. Remain calm.
3. Do not eat or drink anything.

Syndrome X

Syndrome X is not really a specific disease so much as it is a group of conditions that often appear together. Generally, syndrome X, often referred to as the metabolic syndrome, indicates the combination of high blood pressure (hypertension), high lipid levels (LDL cholesterol, triglycerides and other blood fats), obesity (especially around the abdomen), and some form of insulin resistance, though there are varying definitions. People with this combination of risk factors run a much higher risk of developing heart disease and full-blown diabetes. If you already have type 2 diabetes, then it is very likely that you have at least some of the other conditions associated with this syndrome, putting you at an even greater risk of serious complications. With the metabolic syndrome, it can be just a matter of time before something more serious comes along.

WHO HAS SYNDROME X?

Too many people, unfortunately. Syndrome X is very common and may affect as much as 25% of the middle-aged population in this country. Although it affects some populations more than others, it tends to be more common among men and minority populations, especially Mexican Americans. As expected, the older you get, the more likely you are to develop the conditions that make up the metabolic syndrome.

WHAT TO DO

Since they are similar, and often appear together, the methods used to treat syndrome X and type 2 diabetes are very similar. The focus is on treating the underlying problems that are causing the conditions to appear—usually poor diet and lack of exercise. If you believe you meet the criteria for the metabolic syndrome, your first step should be to discuss the situation with your doctor or another member of your health care team. They will be able to develop a treatment plan that is right for you. More than likely this plan will include:

• Exercise

• A healthy meal plan, with less cholesterol and more fiber

• Smoking cessation (quitting smoking)

• Hypertension medication, such as ACE inhibitors (if needed)

• Diabetes medications (if needed)

Because obesity is thought to be the main factor contributing to syndrome X, losing weight will be the focus of your treatment. Losing just a few pounds can have a dramatic effect on your health.

The thing to keep in mind is that having the metabolic syndrome puts you at a much greater risk of heart disease, heart attack, and stroke; but it doesn't necessarily mean you will develop heart problems. This is up to you. With exercise and good diet, you can do a lot to counterbalance the negative effects of syndrome X.

Type 1 Diabetes

n type 1 diabetes, your body stops making insulin or makes only a tiny amount. When this happens, you need to take insulin to live and to be healthy.

Without insulin, glucose cannot get into your cells. (Your cells need to burn glucose for energy.) Glucose collects in the blood. Over time, high levels of glucose in the blood may hurt your eyes, kidneys, nerves, heart, and blood vessels.

Type 1 diabetes occurs most often in people under age 30. But it can occur at any age. The signs of type 1 diabetes can come on suddenly and be severe.

SIGNS OF TYPE 1 DIABETES

Frequent urination	Fatigue
Constant hunger	Edginess
Constant thirst	Mood changes
Weight loss	Nausea
Weakness	Vomiting

CAUSES OF TYPE 1 DIABETES

No one knows for sure why people get type 1 diabetes. Some people are born with genes that make them more likely to get it. But many other people with those same genes do not get diabetes. Something else inside or outside the body triggers the disease. Experts don't know what that something is yet. But they are trying to find out.

Most people with type 1 diabetes have high levels of autoantibodies in their blood sometime before they are first diagnosed with the disease. Antibodies are proteins your body makes to destroy bacteria or viruses. Autoantibodies are antibodies that have "gone bad." They attack your body's own tissues. In these people who get type 1 diabetes, autoantibodies may attack insulin or the cells that make insulin.

TREATMENT OF TYPE 1 DIABETES

There is no cure for diabetes. But there are things you can do to live well and care for type 1 diabetes. The things you do to care for your diabetes help you bring blood glucose levels within your range.

1. Take insulin. Insulin injections or an insulin pump replace the insulin you no longer make. Insulin lets your cells take in glucose.

2. Follow a healthy meal plan (see Healthy Eating; and Meal Planning).

3. Stay physically active. Being active helps your cells take in glucose.

4. Check your blood glucose and urine ketones. Self-checks help you keep track of how well your diabetes care plan is working.

5. Get regular checkups. Your health care team can help you make any needed changes in your diabetes care plan.

WHAT ABOUT WIDE SWINGS IN BLOOD GLUCOSE?

Some people with type 1 diabetes have wide, unpredictable swings in blood glucose. This occurs because their bodies have exaggerated responses to food, medication, and stress.

Food is not absorbed in the same amount of time every time you eat. Insulin is also absorbed at different rates. Stress creates the release of different amounts of stress hormones at different times. These things can work alone or together to cause wide swings in blood glucose levels.

If you have wide swings in your blood glucose levels, examine with your health care team your insulin dose, injection technique, site, depth, and timing. You may need to keep careful records for awhile until you can figure out what is causing those extreme highs and lows.

Type 2 Diabetes

n type 2 diabetes, your body does not make enough insulin, or has trouble using the insulin, or both. A person with type 2 diabetes might inject insulin but does not depend on it to live.

If there is not enough insulin or if it's not working right, your cells cannot use the glucose in your blood to make energy. Instead, glucose stays in the blood. This can lead to high blood glucose levels. Over time, high blood glucose levels may hurt your eyes, kidneys, nerves, heart, and blood vessels.

Most people who get type 2 diabetes are over 40 years old. However, it is occurring with increasing frequency in younger populations—even children. Often, there are no signs of the disease.

SIGNS OF TYPE 2 DIABETES

Frequent urination	Tingling or numb hands or feet
Constant thirst	Fatigue
Constant hunger	Weakness
Dry, itchy skin	Infections of the skin, gums, bladder, or vagina that keep coming back or heal slowly
Blurred vision	

CAUSES OF TYPE 2 DIABETES

Experts don't know for sure what causes type 2 diabetes. They do know that you cannot catch it from someone else, like the flu. They also know it is not caused by eating too much sugar. It does run in families. If other members of your family have type 2 diabetes, you are more likely to get it. But it usually takes something else to bring on the disease.

For many people with diabetes, being overweight brings it on. When you are overweight, your body has a harder time using the insulin that it makes. This is called *insulin resistance*. In insulin resistance, your pancreas keeps making insulin to lower blood glucose, but your body does not respond to the insulin as it should. After years of this, your pancreas may just burn out.

TREATMENT OF TYPE 2 DIABETES

There is no cure for diabetes. But there are things you can do to live well and treat it yourself. At first, eating healthier foods and doing more exercise or activity may help you lose weight.

Losing weight may help you get your blood glucose levels into a more normal range and help your body use the insulin it has. If this does not bring your blood glucose levels down to where you want them, you may need to take diabetes pills.

Diabetes pills are drugs that lower blood glucose levels. They are not insulin. If eating healthier foods, increasing activity, and taking diabetes pills do not lower your blood glucose enough, you may need to add insulin. Or you may need to use insulin instead of diabetes pills.

To find out how your treatments are working, there are two things you can do: 1) check your blood glucose levels and 2) have regular medical checkups.

Urine/Blood Ketone Test

Ketones are waste products that are made when your body burns stored fat for energy. Your body burns fat when it can't get glucose to use for energy. This can happen in people with type 1 diabetes for the following reasons:

High glucose. High glucose means you have too much glucose and not enough insulin in your blood. Your body needs insulin to use glucose for energy. If you don't have enough insulin, your body starts to burn fat for energy.

Exercise. When you exercise, your body needs lots of energy. If you don't have enough insulin or enough glucose when you exercise, your body will burn too much fat.

Stress. It may be a physical stress, such as surgery. Or it may be a mental stress, such as an exam. Whatever kind of stress you're under, your body needs energy to handle it. Your body needs so much energy that it will burn fat if you don't have enough glucose.

Illness. You may have a cold, a sore throat, a fever, or an infection. You may have diarrhea or an upset stomach. When you are sick, your body needs extra energy to fight it. Your body may get some of that extra energy from fat.

Pregnancy. When you are pregnant, your body needs to provide energy for two. If you are not eating enough, your body may turn to fat for the energy it needs.

WHAT KETONES CAN DO TO YOUR BODY

If your body burns too much fat too quickly, high levels of ketones can build up in your blood. Ketones make your blood more acidic. Acidic blood upsets your body's chemical balance. Ketones are passed into your urine.

If blood glucose is high, glucose also passes into your urine. Glucose makes your urine thick. Your body pulls fluid from everywhere to thin out the urine. You make lots of urine. You can get dehydrated.

If you are dehydrated and your ketones are high, you may get ketoacidosis. This is life-threatening. Ketoacidosis can develop in as little as 6 hours.

Most people who get ketoacidosis have type 1 diabetes. But everyone with diabetes needs to be alert for the signs of it.

SIGNS OF KETOACIDOSIS

Dry mouth	Dry, flushed skin
Great thirst	Fever
Fruity breath	Fatigue
Loss of appetite	Drowsiness
Stomach pain	Frequent urination
Nausea	Labored breathing
Vomiting	

URINE/BLOOD TEST FOR KETONES

If you have signs of ketoacidosis or are ill, pregnant, or under stress, check your urine or blood for ketones. Check also if your blood glucose is above 250 mg/dl, especially if you are going to exercise.

Urine and/or blood ketone test kits are available at your local pharmacy. You don't need a prescription. Follow the directions provided in the package. Go over the correct way to check with your diabetes care provider.

Most urine tests go like this:

1. Dip the test strip or tape in a sample of your urine, OR urinate on the test strip or tape, OR put drops of urine on the tablet.
2. Wait to see if the tape, strip, or tablet changes color. The directions will tell you how long to wait. You may need to wait anywhere from 10 seconds to 2 minutes.
3. Match the tape, strip, or tablet color to the color chart provided.
4. Record your results. You should record the type of test, the date and time, the result, and anything unusual. For example, maybe you forgot to take your insulin.

Blood ketone test

Blood ketone tests are very similar to glucose tests. Most times you merely apply a drop of blood to a testing strip, which has been placed in the meter, and then read the results.

What to do with the results

If the result shows trace or small amounts of ketones

1. Drink a glass of water every hour.
2. Check blood glucose and ketones every 3 or 4 hours. If blood glucose and ketone numbers are not going down after two checks, call your doctor.

If the result shows moderate or large amounts of ketones

1. Call your doctor right away! Don't wait. If you wait, your ketone levels may go higher.

Vegetarian Diets

Vegetarian diets are based on plant foods. Plant foods include fruits, vegetables, grains, legumes (beans, peas, and lentils), nuts, and seeds. Plant foods have no cholesterol. Most are low in fat and calories. All are high in fiber, vitamins, and minerals.

A vegetarian diet can be a healthy choice for people with diabetes. Vegetarians are less likely to be overweight, to have high cholesterol levels, or to have high blood pressure. Vegetarians are less likely to get heart disease, blood vessel damage, colon or lung cancer, or osteoporosis.

People with type 1 diabetes who become vegetarians may need less insulin. People with type 2 diabetes who become vegetarians may lose weight. Losing weight may improve blood glucose control.

WILL I GET ENOUGH PROTEIN?

Many people who think about eating a vegetarian diet wonder whether they will get enough protein. But there is little need to worry. Most vegetarians are able to get all the protein they need from high-protein grains, legumes, nuts, and seeds. Other vegetarians also get protein from certain animal foods, such as low-fat dairy products, fish, shellfish, and poultry.

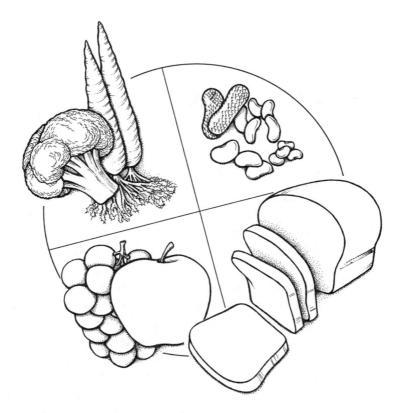

A healthy meal plan contains foods from different groups.

TYPES OF VEGETARIANS

Whether a vegetarian eats animal foods depends on the kind of vegetarian he or she is. There are five kinds of vegetarians: vegan, lacto-vegetarian, ovo-vegetarian, lacto-ovo-vegetarian, and semi-vegetarian. See the table that follows to find out what each kind of vegetarian eats.

TYPES OF VEGETARIANS

Type	Eats	Does Not Eat
Vegan	Fruits, vegetables, legumes, grains, nuts, seeds	Meat, fish, shellfish, poultry, dairy products, eggs
Lacto-Vegetarian	Fruits, vegetables, legumes, grains, nuts, seeds, dairy products	Meat, fish, shellfish, poultry, eggs
Ovo-Vegetarian	Fruits, vegetables, legumes, grains, nuts, seeds, eggs	Meat, fish, shellfish, poultry, dairy products
Lacto-Ovo-Vegetarian	Fruits, vegetables, legumes, grains, nuts, seeds, eggs, dairy products	Meat, fish, shellfish, poultry
Semi-Vegetarian	Fruits, vegetables, legumes, grains, nuts, seeds, eggs, dairy products, fish, shellfish, poultry	Meat

TRYING A VEGETARIAN DIET

If you would like to try a vegetarian diet, talk with a dietitian. A dietitian can help you substitute foods for those you want to take out of your meal plan. A dietitian can help you make sure you get all the nutrients—vitamins, minerals, protein, fats, and carbohydrates—that your body needs. Here are a few suggestions for "going vegetarian."

- Start by eating one vegetarian meal a week for several weeks. Stick with familiar foods at first, such as spaghetti with marinara sauce.

- Read vegetarian cookbooks for recipe ideas.

- Try eating out at a vegetarian restaurant. You may be surprised by the variety of tasty dishes you'll find.

- Eat less meat, poultry, fish, and shellfish in your meals. An ideal portion is 3 oz—about the size of a deck of cards.

- Cut meat into cubes or strips and add to a salad or grain dish.
- Eat more grains, legumes, and vegetables in your meals.
- Try cooked beans in place of some of the meat in your chili, stir-fries, stews, and casseroles.
- Remember that replacing meat with vegetable proteins, such as beans, will increase the amount of carbohydrates you eat. Make sure you test your blood sugar and work with your physician and dietitian during the process.

Vitamins and Minerals

The right amounts of vitamins and minerals help your body function well. You can get vitamins and minerals from the foods you eat. You can also get vitamins and minerals from pills. These are called supplements.

Most people with diabetes get enough vitamins and minerals by eating a variety of foods. Some people with diabetes may be deficient in certain vitamins and minerals. Being deficient means your body does not have enough of a vitamin or mineral.

VITAMIN DEFICIENCIES

Most people with diabetes get enough vitamin A. Most people with diabetes also get enough vitamin E and vitamin C, but a few people may need more. Check with your doctor about this.

People with diabetes usually get enough of the B vitamins. The B vitamins include vitamin B_1 (thiamin), vitamin B_2 (riboflavin), vitamin B_3 (niacin), vitamin B_6 (pyridoxine), vitamin B_{12}, and folate. If your diabetes is in poor control, though, you risk losing the B vitamins in your urine. Your diabetes care provider may advise you to eat more foods high in the B vitamins.

Research has shown that a deficiency in vitamin B_6 may be related to impaired glucose tolerance. Impaired glucose tolerance means your body has a hard time using insulin.

FOOD SOURCES OF VITAMINS AND MINERALS

Vitamin A	Liver, tuna, deep-orange fruits and vegetables, leafy greens
Vitamin B$_1$ (thiamin)	Pork, sunflower seeds, whole grains
Vitamin B$_2$ (riboflavin)	Liver, duck, mackerel, dairy foods
Vitamin B$_3$ (niacin)	Poultry, fish, veal
Vitamin B$_6$ (pyridoxine)	Potatoes, bananas, chickpeas, prune juice, poultry, fish, liver
Vitamin B$_{12}$	Fish, shellfish, liver
Vitamin C	Citrus fruits, melon, strawberries, kiwifruit, bell peppers, broccoli, Brussels sprouts
Vitamin D	Fish, fortified milk, butter, margarine, eggs
Vitamin E	Nuts, seeds, oils, mangos, blackberries, apples
Folate	Legumes, leafy greens, asparagus, liver, wheat germ
Calcium	Yogurt, milk, cheese
Chromium	Wheat germ, brewer's yeast, bran, whole grains, liver, meats, cheese
Copper	Crab, liver, nuts, seeds, prunes, raisins
Iron	Shellfish, meats, liver, soybeans, pumpkin seeds
Magnesium	Nuts, seeds, legumes, whole grains, leafy greens, fish
Manganese	Whole grains, vegetables, nuts, fruits
Potassium	Fruits, vegetables, legumes, fish, milk, yogurt
Selenium	Shellfish, fish, liver, nuts, whole grains
Zinc	Meats, liver, shellfish

MINERAL DEFICIENCIES

Chromium. Most people with diabetes get enough chromium. But a few people with diabetes have a chromium deficiency. A chromium deficiency can cause higher blood glucose and blood fat levels and impaired glucose tolerance.

If a lab test shows that you have a chromium deficiency, your doctor may have you take a chromium supplement. If you already get enough chromium, taking extra will not help your blood glucose or blood fat levels.

Copper and manganese. Deficiencies in copper and manganese have been linked to impaired glucose tolerance. But most people with diabetes get enough copper and manganese. So deficiencies are not likely.

Selenium and iron. Deficiencies in selenium in people with diabetes are not likely. And most people with diabetes are not at any greater risk for iron deficiency than people without diabetes.

Magnesium. People with diabetes who have poor blood glucose control or have very high ketones are more likely to become deficient in magnesium. A lack of magnesium may make your body less sensitive to insulin. If a lab test shows that your magnesium level is low, your doctor may have you take magnesium supplements.

Zinc. Deficiencies in zinc are more likely in people with diabetes, especially those in poor control. Lack of zinc may cause impaired glucose tolerance. If a lab test shows you do not have enough zinc, your doctor may have you take a supplement or eat more foods high in zinc.

VITAMIN OR MINERAL SUPPLEMENTS

Check with your health care team to be sure you are getting the vitamins and minerals you need. If your team finds that you lack some vitamins and minerals, they may recommend a supplement.

If you are trying to lose weight and take in fewer than 1,200 calories each day

You may need iron and folate.

If you eat no animal foods at all

You may need vitamin B_{12}, calcium, iron, vitamin B_2 (riboflavin), and zinc.

If you are at risk for bone diseases

You may need vitamin D, calcium, and magnesium.

If you are over 65 years old

You may need calcium and folate.

If you are pregnant or breastfeeding

You may need extra iron, zinc, calcium, and folate.

If you take diuretics (water pills)

You may need magnesium, calcium, potassium, and zinc.

Check with your doctor before taking any supplement.

THE RIGHT DOSE

The National Academy of Sciences establishes Recommended Dietary Allowances (RDAs) and Safe and Adequate Intakes for vitamins and minerals. These are the minimum amounts of vitamins and minerals that most people need. Healthy people with diabetes need to get these amounts.

RECOMMENDED DIETARY ALLOWANCES OR SAFE AND ADEQUATE INTAKES OF VITAMINS AND MINERALS FOR MEN AND WOMEN AGED 25 TO 50 YEARS

	Men	Women
Vitamin A	1,000 μg RE	800 μg RE
Vitamin B$_1$ (thiamin)	1.5 mg	1.1 mg
Vitamin B$_2$ (riboflavin)	1.7 mg	1.3 mg
Vitamin B$_3$ (niacin)	19 mg	15 mg
Vitamin B$_6$ (pyridoxine)	2 mg	1.6 mg
Vitamin B$_{12}$	2.0 μg	2.0 μg
Vitamin C	60 mg	60 mg
Vitamin D	5 μg	5 μg
Vitamin E	10 mg αTE	8 mg αTE
Folate	200 μg	180 μg
Calcium	800 mg	800 mg
Chromium	50 to 200 μg	50 to 200 μg
Copper	1.5 to 3.0 mg	1.5 to 3.0 mg
Iron	10 mg	15 mg
Magnesium	350 mg	280 mg
Manganese	2.0 to 5.0 mg	2.0 to 5.0 mg
Potassium	3,500 mg	3,500 mg
Selenium	70 μg	55 μg
Zinc	15 mg	12 mg

RE stands for retinol equivalents. Since 1974, the National Academy of Sciences has been using retinol equivalents (RE) instead of international units (I.U.) to measure vitamin A in food for vitamin A requirements. αTE stands for alpha-tocopherol equivalents. Alpha-tocopherol is the most easily absorbed form of vitamin E.

Weight Loss

f you are overweight, losing weight is one of the best treatments for type 2 diabetes. Losing weight will lower your blood pressure, lower your risk of heart disease and blood vessel damage, and improve your blood glucose control.

Your blood glucose control may improve so much that you can cut down on your insulin or diabetes pills. Sometimes, losing just 10 pounds is enough to improve diabetes control.

Your health care team can help you decide how much weight loss would be good for you. They can also help you make a weight-loss plan. Your plan will include a weight-loss goal. Break down your goal into smaller goals that you can easily meet. You may set weekly or monthly weight-loss goals.

When you meet a smaller goal, reward yourself with a book, a CD, an outing, or a piece of clothing, for example. Once you have set your goals, you are ready to start your weight-loss program.

The only way to lose weight is to eat less and exercise more. And the only way to keep the weight off is to keep up these two new habits for the rest of your healthy life.

WAYS TO EAT LESS

"Eat less" actually means "eat fewer calories." You may need to eat smaller portions. Or, you may be able to eat the same amount of food, if you eat foods that are lower in calories.

Fat has more than twice as many calories as carbohydrate or protein. So if you eat less fat and more carbohydrate and protein, you will get fewer calories. For more on eating this way, see Healthy Eating.

Food tips

- Serve food from the stove. Leave the food there instead of putting it on the table. Going for seconds won't be as easy.
- Eat slowly and stop when you just begin to feel full. That way, you won't get too full.
- Don't watch TV, read, or listen to the radio while you eat. These activities may draw your attention away from how much you are eating and whether you are full.
- Ask another family member to put leftovers away. That way, you won't be tempted to eat the remaining food.
- Brush your teeth right after you eat. This gets the taste of food out of your mouth and may get the thought of food out of your head.
- Don't go grocery shopping when you are hungry. You may buy too much. Or you may buy things that aren't on your meal plan.
- Write out a grocery list before you go shopping. Buy just what is on the list.
- Store food out of sight.
- Eat something before you go to a social function. That way, you'll be less likely to overeat fatty foods.
- Don't skip a meal. You may overeat at your next one.
- Don't forbid yourself to eat certain foods. You'll only want them more. Try to cut down on the size of the serving or the number of times you eat that food in a week.

WAYS TO EXERCISE MORE

Exercise takes weight off by helping you burn calories. If you exercise regularly, your muscles will continue to burn calories even while you're at rest.

Different exercises burn different numbers of calories. Some good exercises for weight loss are cross-country skiing, walking, swimming, bicycling, and low-impact aerobics.

It's best to exercise at a moderate pace so you can keep going for a long time. If you exercise at a high pace, you will tire yourself out before you have a chance to burn enough calories. The longer you exercise, the more calories you burn.

You might start with a 5-minute walk each day. Add 5 minutes to the walk at the beginning of the week. Build up to where you can walk for 45 to 60 minutes. Try to do that four or more times a week.

To burn even more calories, add physical activities throughout the day. Walk, don't drive. Take the stairs, not the elevator. Spend the night out bowling or dancing instead of watching TV. For more ideas on increasing your physical activity, see Activity.

Motivating tips

- Choose exercises and activities that you enjoy.
- Pick a convenient time and place for your exercise or activity.
- Select an exercise or activity that's within your financial budget.
- Don't worry about your weight. You will replace fat tissue with muscle. Muscle weighs more than fat.
- Check your measurements with a tape measure. You'll be able to see that you're getting leaner.

HOW TO KEEP THE WEIGHT OFF

When you have reached your body weight goal, the hard part comes. Keeping weight off is much more difficult than losing it.

Most people will regain lost weight. Many people gain back even more weight than they lost. This happens because people return to their old eating and exercise habits after they lose weight.

You will need to keep up your new eating and exercise habits to stay at your goal body weight. The trade off is that you'll probably look and feel better.

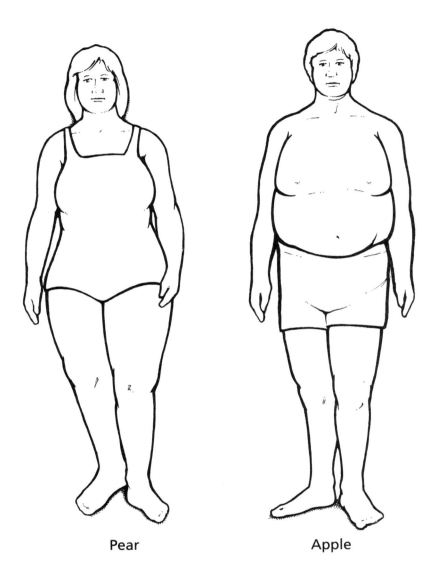

Pear   Apple

People who carry more weight on the hips and thighs are pear-shaped. People who carry more weight around the waist and abdomen are apple-shaped. Apple-shaped people are more likely to have blood vessel damage, heart disease, high blood pressure, high blood fat levels, insulin resistance, and poor blood glucose control.

Yoga

Staying active is a big part of controlling your blood glucose levels with diabetes, especially type 2 diabetes. It seems that every year, more and more research shows that exercise and activity can go a long way toward helping your body use insulin more efficiently. In fact, some believe that exercise might be one of the most important factors in keeping blood glucose levels near normal.

There are many forms of exercise and countless ways to stay active. These range from weeding the garden to taking a walk to riding cross-country on a bicycle. There are also different ways to focus your activity to get different results. You can concentrate on building strength with resistance activities, such as lifting weights. You can focus on elevating your heart rate for a period of time with aerobic exercises, such as jogging. You can also focus on increasing your flexibility with stretching exercises, such as yoga.

YOGA AND FLEXIBILITY

Flexibility is a part of exercise that is often overlooked. Many people tend to focus on building muscles or improving their aerobic capacity. Stretching and flexibility is usually seen as something you do before you exercise, not as exercise in its own right. However, improving your flexibility through activities such as yoga can reap a lot of rewards.

Flexibility is generally thought of as how far you can comfortably move your muscles around your joints, or your range of motion. Being able to stretch your muscles is good because it:

- Decreases tension on your muscles

- Helps prevent injury

- Eases muscle and joint discomfort

Yoga is an excellent way to improve flexibility because it works stretching exercises into a complete, low-impact, full-body program. It involves holding your body in various positions or doing a series of slow movements while you concentrate on your breathing patterns. Yoga is an excellent choice if you haven't been active for a while, you're recovering from an injury, or you have limited mobility. It's also a good addition to any cross-training routine, since it works muscles you don't normally use. In addition to improving your flexibility, yoga also:

- Increases strength

- Increases energy

- Relieves physical and mental stress

There are many different types of yoga (some more active, others more meditative), so be sure to look into the various choices to find the type that is right for you. Generally, it's also better to take a yoga class, as opposed to following a book or tape. Having a yoga instructor there to make sure you are in the correct position and doing the exercises correctly can be a big help.

Yoga may not be right for everyone. If you have high blood pressure or retinopathy, you should not place your head below your waist. Before you begin any new exercise program, discuss the activity with your doctor or a member of your health care team. Not only will they be able to assess your ability to take part in an activity such as yoga, but they will also be able to provide you with information on local groups, classes, and other resources.

Zzz's—Sleep Is Important

A mericans are a severely sleep deprived people. Adults in this country, on average, sleep only 6 1/2 hours a night, with a third of us sleeping even less than that. Fifty years ago, people averaged an hour more sleep than we do today. Eighty years ago, people got about 2 hours more. So why can't we sleep? Nobody can pinpoint one single reason, but some suspect it is too much work, too much stress, too much TV and Internet, or a combination of all three. Whatever the reason, there seems to be something keeping us from getting a good night's rest.

The effects of not having enough sleep can be very harmful. Besides just making us less alert in our daily lives (some studies suggest that 10% of all auto accidents and most job-related accidents are caused by fatigue), being sleep deprived can disrupt the way your body works to regulate itself. Lack of sleep has been linked to high blood pressure, heart attack, and stroke. Recent research suggests that not getting enough sleep can even cause diabetes, or for those who already have diabetes, cause complications from diabetes to worsen.

SLEEP AND DIABETES

How can lack of sleep cause diabetes? While the cause is still not known, it appears that sleep helps regulate certain hormones that work together to determine how sensitive you are to insulin. When you do not get enough sleep, your body becomes less sensitive to insulin. In one study of sleep-deprived young males, insulin levels in the blood were up to

50% higher when they did not get enough sleep. It may not always be this striking, but not getting enough sleep appears to be directly linked to high levels of insulin in the bloodstream. Over time, these high levels of insulin can cause your body to become more and more insulin resistant, and possibly lead to diabetes.

If you already have diabetes, the effects of too little sleep can be even more dramatic. The insulin resistance that comes with not enough sleep can intensify your preexisting diabetes, making it much harder to control your blood glucose levels and putting you at a much higher risk of developing complications. If you have diabetes or are at risk for diabetes, getting enough sleep is not just a matter of being better rested, it's a matter of good health.

Sleep apnea

Getting a good night's sleep is easier said than done, however. In addition to the many lifestyle obstacles that often keep us from getting enough sleep—stress, entertainment, and insomnia—people with diabetes often suffer from a sleeping disorder call *sleep apnea*. Sleep apnea prevents people from getting enough oxygen while they sleep, which can interrupt deep sleep and make it harder to get good rest. Most people with sleep apnea aren't aware that they suffer from the disorder, and it has been suggested that 9 out of 10 people with sleep apnea go undiagnosed. If you have sleep apnea, you may often feel very tired, even after many hours of sleep, and have trouble getting out of bed in the morning. Although a link has not been clearly established, sleep apnea, diabetes, and obesity often go hand in hand.

Besides keeping you from feeling rested, sleep apnea can produce the same insulin-resistant effects that come from not getting enough sleep. It has been suggested that just like lack of sleep in general, there's a link between sleep apnea and an increased rate of heart disease, heart attack, and stroke, though this may not be caused by sleep apnea; the two conditions may just be caused by a common source.

Fortunately, there are treatments for sleep apnea that can be very effective. If you feel you suffer from this condition, talk with a member of your diabetes care team about what treatments might be right for you.

TIPS FOR GOOD SLEEP

- Reserve the bed for sleep (and intimacy) only. Doing other activities in bed, such as watching TV, discussing emotional issues, or working on a laptop, can cause you to associate the bed with things other than sleep.

- Avoid naps in the afternoon or early evening.

- Avoid caffeine, nicotine (don't smoke!), and alcohol in the evening. Alcohol may seem as if it helps put you to sleep, but as it is processed by your body, it can cause you to wake early and may cause nightmares and sweats.

- Try to establish a calming, pre-bed ritual. It can often be hard to "turn off" the stresses of daily life and simply fall asleep. Performing a calming activity before you go to sleep, such as taking a hot bath, meditating, or listening to calming music, will help clear your mind of the stress of daily life.

- Minimize bright lights, noise, and other aggravating factors in your sleep area.

- A light snack before bed can be relaxing (and, if you take insulin, help avoid nighttime lows), but a full meal right before you go to bed can make it hard to sleep.

- Try to go to sleep and wake at the same time every day, even on weekends. Getting your body into a sleeping rhythm is very important.

- If you feel you have a sleeping disorder, such as sleep apnea, insomnia, or narcolepsy, talk with your health care team about options for treatment.

Index

About the American Diabetes Association

The American Diabetes Association is the nation's leading voluntary health organization supporting diabetes research, information, and advocacy. Its mission is to prevent and cure diabetes and to improve the lives of all people affected by diabetes. The American Diabetes Association is the leading publisher of comprehensive diabetes information. Its huge library of practical and authoritative books for people with diabetes covers every aspect of self-care—cooking and nutrition, fitness, weight control, medications, complications, emotional issues, and general self-care.

To order American Diabetes Association books: Call 1-800-232-6733. Or log on to http://store.diabetes.org

To join the American Diabetes Association: Call 1-800-806-7801. www.diabetes.org/membership

For more information about diabetes or ADA programs and services: Call 1-800-342-2383. E-mail: AskADA@diabetes.org or log on to www.diabetes.org

To locate an ADA/NCQA Recognized Provider of quality diabetes care in your area: www.ncqa.org/dprp/

To find an ADA Recognized Education Program in your area: Call 1-888-232-0822. www.diabetes.org/recognition/education.asp

To join the fight to increase funding for diabetes research, end discrimination, and improve insurance coverage: Call 1-800-342-2383. www.diabetes.org/advocacy

To find out how you can get involved with the programs in your community: Call 1-800-342-2383. See below for program Web addresses.

- *Diabetes Month:* Educational activities aimed at those diagnosed with diabetes—month of November. www.diabetes.org/ADM
- *American Diabetes Alert:* Annual public awareness campaign to find the undiagnosed—held the fourth Tuesday in March. www.diabetes.org/alert
- *The Diabetes Assistance & Resources Program (DAR):* diabetes awareness program targeted to the Latino community. www.diabetes.org/DAR
- *African American Program:* diabetes awareness program targeted to the African American community. www.diabetes.org/africanamerican
- *Awakening the Spirit: Pathways to Diabetes Prevention & Control:* diabetes awareness program targeted to the Native American community. www.diabetes.org/awakening

To find out about an important research project regarding type 2 diabetes: www.diabetes.org/ada/research.asp

To obtain information on making a planned gift or charitable bequest: Call 1-888-700-7029. www.diabetes.org/ada/plan.asp

To make a donation or memorial contribution: Call 1-800-342-2383. www.diabetes.org/ada/cont.asp